Reverse
Heart Disease
Now

Reverse Heart Disease Now

Stop Deadly Cardiovascular Plaque
Before It's Too Late

STEPHEN SINATRA, M.D., F.A.C.C.,
and
JAMES C. ROBERTS, M.D., F.A.C.C.,

with Martin Zucker

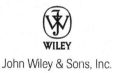

WILEY

John Wiley & Sons, Inc.

Published by John Wiley & Sons, Inc., Hoboken, New Jersey
Published simultaneously in Canada

Illustrations by Linda Tenukas

Design and composition by Navta Associates, Inc.

The information contained in this book is not intended to serve as a replacement for professional medical advice. Any use of the information in this book is at the reader's discretion. The author and the publisher specifically disclaim any and all liability arising directly or indirectly from the use or application of any information contained in this book. A health care professional should be consulted regarding your specific situation.

Designations used by companies to distinguish their products are often claimed as trademarks. In all instances where John Wiley & Sons, Inc., is aware of a claim, the product names appear in Initial Capital or ALL CAPITAL letters. Readers, however, should contact the appropriate companies for more complete information regarding trademarks and registration.

For general information about our other products and services, please contact our Customer Care Department within the United States at (800) 762-2974, outside the United States at (317) 572-3993 or fax (317) 572-4002.

Wiley also publishes its books in a variety of electronic formats. Some content that appears in print may not be available in electronic books. For more information about Wiley products, visit our web site at www.wiley.com.

Library of Congress Cataloging-in-Publication Data:

Sinatra, Stephen T.
    Reverse heart disease now : stop deadly cardiovascular plaque before it's too late / Stephen Sinatra and James Roberts ; with Martin Zucker.
        p. cm.
    Includes bibliographical references and index.
    ISBN: 978-0-471-74704-8 (cloth)
    ISBN: 978-0-470-22878-4 (paper)
    1. Heart—Diseases—Alternative treatment—Popular works. 2. Heart—Diseases—Prevention—Popular works. 3. Atherosclerotic plaque. I.
Roberts, James, date— II. Zucker, Martin. III. Title.
    RC684.A48S564 2006
    616.1'205—dc22

                                                                                    2006004868

Printed in the United States of America

10 9 8 7 6 5 4 3 2 1

To Jan, Cindy, and Rosita—our wives—for their love, patience, and support.

Contents

Preface

From Crisis to Prevention:
The Transformation of Two Cardiologists

We consider ourselves a new breed of cardiologists—making our patients healthier and keeping them out of hospitals. We were once "typical" board-certified cardiologists. We did thousands of angiograms and performed emergency cardiac procedures. We rolled up our sleeves at all hours of the day and night. We did what we were trained to do and thought we did the very best for our patients. We saw ourselves as saviors.

In the beginning, we didn't know there were other ways to practice cardiology other than what we had been taught. Then we learned differently. We learned we could stabilize killer arterial plaque—stop it in its tracks—and maybe even reverse it. And what we learned changed our lives and the lives of our patients.

Independently, something big happened to us both on our journey as cardiologists. Medically speaking, we became born-again doctors with an enlarged vision that transformed the way we practice. We refer to it as New Cardiology or integrative cardiology, and it gives us dynamic tools to raise patients to the highest level of their health potential. It brings together conventional care with complementary care. In this new format, we are as comfortable recommending nutritional supplements and mind/body approaches as we are prescribing bypass surgery or a heart drug. We integrate what works the best.

Over the years, we have seen a slow but growing acceptance within the medical profession regarding the effectiveness of natural alternatives for a wide range of cardiovascular disorders such as angina, arrhythmias, high blood pressure, and heart failure. This is the way it should be: integrating the best of conventional medicine with natural healing.

We believe this is smart medicine that can save countless lives and make a huge dent in the continuing epidemic of cardiovascular disease.

Usually, with a combined program of nutritional medicine, medications, or reverse lifestyle changes, and, if necessary, surgery, we can stabilize or reverse existing disease. Many of our sickest patients make remarkable recoveries.

We have written this book as a guide for you, the medical consumer. It is an effort to explain and demonstrate the benefits of an integrated cardiology approach based on our medical research and our combined fifty years of clinical cardiology practice. The information will help you understand how arteries become enveloped in inflammation and plaque, which may lead to heart attack, stroke, and heart failure.

We also want to show how patients and doctors can work together to promote health and vitality. There are wonderful options—medications and scientifically proven supplements and lifestyle changes—with which to extinguish the flames of disease and promote good blood flow, even for the most compromised cases. This book is about integrating those options to restore and maintain the best possible arterial function and a vigorously pumping heart. It is a guide to improving and saving lives.

Dr. Sinatra's Story

Many years ago, a cardiologist called me to transfer a very sick patient from the emergency room where I was working to another hospital. The patient was too sick to transfer. His blood pressure was way down. He had chest pains. I tried to discourage the doctor, reminding him that the patient was very unstable, it was the middle of winter, and it was four o'clock in the morning. But the patient's wife wanted him transferred. When she finally understood that her husband could die in the ambulance, she turned to me and asked, "Are you any good?" I looked her in the eyes and said, "I'm the best there is," a line I remembered from a Clint Eastwood movie in which he was an ace pilot. That calmed her down. She had to hear that. She accepted the plan that her husband stay put, and happily we were able to help him.

Over the years, I've treated countless cardiac emergencies—people literally a heartbeat away from death. I've done middle-of-the-night heroics and slept in hospital beds next to critical patients. I felt I was the very best in an emergency. I became pompous in the process.

It's hard to put into words all this running from one emergency to another. For four or five years, I never ate lunch. I had no time for it. My lifestyle was very hard on my family life. My beeper would go off in the middle of my son's soccer game. This was before cell phones, and I'd leave to find a pay phone to call the hospital. It was a good life in the sense that I felt I was always needed but a hard life, nevertheless. When I got home from work, I couldn't talk to my wife because I was all wired up and exhausted.

I would go into the hospital at eight in the morning and get home at nine or ten at night. On the weekends, I would make rounds on fifty or more people. I took an enormous amount of night calls and never saw my kids. I felt I was a terrible father because I wasn't available. I can remember one Christmas morning. It was six o'clock. I had a one-year-old and a two-year-old, and I had to rush to the hospital to put in an emergency pacemaker for one of my patients. I left a cup of steaming coffee on the kitchen table and unopened packages under the Christmas tree.

One day, I woke up and seriously questioned what I was doing. I liked my job, but I also hated it.

After doing some heroics on a heart patient whom we had treated before, I told another doctor that we were barking up the wrong tree. We prescribed drugs and applied different therapies aimed at directly fixing the problem. For the short term, our efforts worked. We were doing all the things we were trained to do but we weren't helping to heal our patients for the long term.

Often, we couldn't save people. I vividly remember a case one year out of cardiology specialty training when a man was rushed into the emergency room. We couldn't do anything for him. He was in his early forties. I had to go out and tell his wife that she lost her husband. When our eyes first met, I knew that she knew. She had two blond twins with her, about five years old. That was very hard to do. And I had to do things like that a lot.

In that same year—it was 1978—I encountered Jacob Rinse, a ninety-one-year-old Dutch petroleum chemist who changed my life. Years before, he had been diagnosed with severe coronary artery disease but had refused bypass surgery. Being an inquisitive scientist, he had investigated the nature of heart disease and formulated his own vitamin and mineral concoctions. He thrived on the home-made program.

One of my patients, a particularly difficult case, asked me to contact Rinse for suggestions. During a phone conversation, the chemist told me that he had the secret treatment for atherosclerosis. Being a cocky young cardiologist, I was initially amused, but I soon realized I was talking to somebody who described the chemistry of heart disease in a way I hadn't heard before. He may have been "old" and far removed from the medical world, but he was as sharp as a tack, and his voice resonated with vitality. I listened as he told me about the formula he used to help himself and others who were interested. He described how lecithin, vitamin E, magnesium, and other nutrients could help prevent arterial clogging.

I was taken aback. I had never heard anything like that in medical school or my cardiology training. I began to think that maybe there was more to medicine than just drugs and surgery. That fleeting conversation with Rinse turned the path of my career in the direction of integrative medicine. I still continued my intense work, but I was formulating a different way to deal with heart disease before—and not just after—the heart attack.

I started recommending vitamins E and C and talking about diet and exercise to patients. Over time, I began to see improvement in patients who followed my suggestions. I was so impressed that I went for an advanced degree in nutrition.

In the early 1980s, I learned about CoQ10, a vitamin depleted by poor diet and the aging process. This substance is a major chemical participant in cellular energy production. As such, it's critically important for strong pumping action of the heart. Plus it provides superb protection against arterial plaque formation.

An article in a medical journal had caught my attention. It reported how patients taking CoQ10 were able to be weaned quickly from the heart–lung bypass machine used during open heart surgeries. I had recently lost a dear patient after a successful mitral valve replacement operation because he failed to come off that same pump—a nightmare scenario that happens on rare occasions. The article made a strong impression. What if I had known about CoQ10 before I'd sent that kind man for surgery? His death had hit me hard.

I couldn't bring him back, but I could tell patients awaiting open heart surgery to start taking CoQ10 daily. Those patients have all come off the heart–lung bypass machine without a problem.

All through the 1980s, I found myself driven to learn all I could about mind/body and nutritional medicine. It consumed most of my spare time. I found major healing benefits for my patients using B vitamins, fish oil, green tea, and exciting natural substances with strange names like nattokinase and phospholipids. They transformed sick lives into revived and energized lives. They gave patients the optimism and encouragement to become more involved in their own healing process. They unclogged and defused arteries, revolutionizing my practice from crisis management to crisis prevention and from illness to health.

I saw patients reach levels of healing I could never imagine possible with conventional care alone. Instead of tears of sorrow, I repeatedly witnessed tears of joy. I received hearty hugs from rejuvenated patients.

The idea of stabilizing plaque and even reversing it became my obsession—the challenge of a career. I just had to keep connecting the dots and keeping an open mind to new ideas.

Dr. Roberts's Story

I was a midnight warrior at the start of my cardiology practice. I was in the hospital all the time. There were eight coronary care unit beds in the hospital where I was on staff. One Tuesday afternoon, I was managing all eight patients. I was doing invasive procedures over and over.

In basketball they talk about triple doubles: players striving to reach double digits in scoring points, rebounding, and assisting other scorers in a game. The best players do it maybe a few times in a season. In my work, I strived for a triple double every day. That meant any three of the following "performances": two pacemakers, two angiograms, two right heart catheterizations for heart failure, two balloon pumps, two admissions. That was my big macho thing. I got into the "performance" mode, sucked up into making a lot of money and admitting more patients to the hospital than anybody else. I wanted to be the number one producer and the number one savior. I worked hard and accomplished my goals, and I felt I was the best.

After four or five years in practice, I began to realize that I was falling into a frustrating pattern: treating the same people over and over without really getting them well. The same patients always came back. It was a revolving door. I would do heroics for their heart, but they might develop gastrointestinal tract bleeding or kidney failure as a side effect of the treatment. I felt like I was spinning my wheels.

I would treat someone with heart failure in crisis, a patient short of breath, his or her lungs full of fluid because of a stiff heart not pumping effectively. I would overcome the immediate danger and send the patient home. But because we weren't dealing with the cause of the heart failure, the patient would return in crisis again.

A patient would be rushed in by ambulance with a heart attack, an acute coronary blockage. Our medical team would go into crisis mode, administering a clot-dissolving drug, doing an acute angiogram, dealing with the artery narrowing, and if we were lucky and good, getting the patient over the hump. But we didn't do anything about what made that artery clog. Two years later, the same patient would be back because another artery was clogged or possibly even the same one. After a while, I realized these patients were always going to come back. I realized that unless something changed, my pager would always go off and I would always have to leave before my son got to bat in his Little League games. And I would be sleepless many nights during the rest of my life.

I began to think what if we could just prevent these emergencies in the first place. If we could just prevent the artery from going bad, then we wouldn't have to do middle-of-the-night heroics. There had to be a better way.

I began thinking seriously about prevention and alternatives after encountering several older patients with alarmingly high cholesterol levels but totally normal coronary arteries. They told me they were taking vitamins and they felt that the vitamins were protecting them.

Around this time, a persistent patient hounded me about something called antioxidants. He gave me a research paper to read that contained information about free radicals and antioxidant vitamins—things I hadn't learned in medical school. My eyes opened wide and so did my appetite for more knowledge. What I learned made sense to me. I started putting patients on vitamins C, E, and B complex, magnesium and selenium, and CoQ10.

Within a year, I noticed my hospital admissions dropping. My patients were doing better, and I was starting to feel that I could actually do something besides crisis management.

If the antioxidants worked, I wanted to know what else worked. That led to fish oils. I saw another level of improvement. I felt I was really onto something. I started going to meetings on nutritional medicine. I studied the medical literature on causation of heart disease. As I applied my new knowledge, the crises among my patients became fewer and fewer. I felt exceedingly gratified. I had more time to do prevention. The old patient/new crisis revolving door practically stopped.

New patients would come to me, having heard that there's a doctor in town doing things differently and getting sick patients well. They would often be last-resort cases. Those challenges would spur more digging to learn even more to help them.

Today, I regard a hospital admission as a failure on my part. The hospital nurses who have known me for many years kid me when I admit a patient. Once the top admitter, I'm quite happy now as a distant also-ran.

I still see acutely sick and inoperable people, but I can get them on a program that stabilizes their plaque. That means my sleep is stabilized.

My patients take their necessary medications. That's important and often critical to their survival. But the difference is that they are taking supplements that stop or minimize the damage that ruins their arteries and heart cells. Over a ten-year period, this approach has totally revolutionized my practice.

Acknowledgments

To Jan Sinatra, as always, for sharing ideas and encouragement, and for giving our manuscript a sharp-eyed but caring review.

To Jo-Anne Piazza, invaluable assistant, adviser, and confidante, whose cheerful coordinating and research skills helped ensure productive, seamless interactions between multiple authors.

To Ralph E. Holsworth, Jr., D.O., of Pagosa Springs, Colorado, for sharing his unique experience with nattokinase, an amazing nutritional supplement.

To Richard M. Delany, M.D., F.A.C.C., of Milton, Massachusetts, a fellow traveler in the frontier of New Cardiology. Thank you for sharing your perspective on the potential of genetic testing.

To Paul H. Keyes, D.S.S., the esteemed dental researcher who years ago helped uncover the bacterial connection of caries and periodontal disease, which we now know can spread inflammation and disease to the cardiovascular system.

To Thomas Miller, Teryn Kendall, and Kimberly Monroe-Hill, our editors, for sound, practical advice on how to unclog a weighty manuscript, making it lean and more reader-friendly.

To Anna Ghosh and Jack Scovil, our agents at Scovil Chichak Galen Literary Agency in New York, for steady steerage through contractual issues.

To Linda Tenukas, our talented and rapid-response illustrator.

Introduction

The New Cardiology

In 1977, Joe was experiencing chest pain. The quality of his life was poor. To manage his pain, he was chewing on nitroglycerin tablets daily.

Dr. Sinatra performed an angiogram. Joe's major coronary arteries looked like rosary beads full of plaque pockets. They were so blocked that the surgeon could not find a place to implant a bypass graft, although he would have tried if there had been no other options. Because Joe's heart rate was so low, a pacemaker was inserted. With the pacemaker, beta blockers, and nitroglycerine, his chest pain improved.

In 1980, Joe read about intravenous chelation, an alternative therapy for cardiovascular disease that removes harmful substances such as lead, cadmium, and arsenic from the body. Dr. Sinatra suggested this therapy, so Joe had sixty intravenous (IV) chelation treatments. His overall health improved, but he still had recurrent bouts of angina. He was still taking nitroglycerin but less, and continued to be helped by the pacemaker.

During the next few years, Dr. Sinatra put Joe on a multivitamin, mineral, and antioxidant supplement program, and then on coenzyme Q10 (CoQ10). In 1987, Joe had another angiogram because of recalcitrant chest pains. One of the coronary arteries showed no progression of disease, another showed regression, and another some progression. From a physician's perspective, it was phenomenal that Joe was still alive, let alone doing this well. Sixty percent of people in his condition die within five years. Clearly, the disease was more stable, but the progression in one vessel indicated he still needed help.

In the early 1990s, the amino acid L-carnitine was added to the program to support the action of CoQ10. Joe also did another round of thirty IV chelation treatments. He did exceedingly well. He was walking farther and taking less medication.

In the mid-1990s, Joe was walking two miles a day, but he still experienced some angina from time to time and had to stop to rest.

In the late 1990s, a fish oil supplement was added to his regimen. He improved again. But still there was some stubborn shortness of breath.

In 2004, Joe added D-ribose and nattokinase, two cutting-edge supplements, and improved even more.

To a cardiologist, this is a miracle. Today, Joe is in his nineties and doing great, a spiritual patient with a positive attitude. He exercises and eats a healthy diet. He is a model patient who has done everything asked of him. And all this has made a huge impact on his quality of life and longevity. Now he takes a minimum amount of medication. He takes nitroglycerin only on an as-needed basis, mostly in the winter when the cold weather causes the angina because his heart has to work harder.

Dr. Sinatra feels that the next time he sees Joe, there will be something else to add to the program and notch up his well-being even more.

Integrate, Not Separate

Joe's story represents the power of integrative medicine and, we believe, the future of cardiology.

When we see patients for the first time, it is often because their cardiologist has told them to stop taking vitamins and they're confused. Some doctors are often uncomfortable with their patients taking supplements. In most cases, it's fear of the unknown. They haven't been trained to use supplements, so they aren't sufficiently familiar, and therefore usually dismiss them. The dismissive attitude shortchanges patients, because today so much scientific evidence validates the potentially lifesaving benefits of many nutritional supplements.

On the other side of the medical practice spectrum, doctors who offer only alternative therapies to patients with very sick hearts may be foolishly denying them the full range of effective care. Such was the case of Janet, a patient who required urgent coronary artery bypass surgery.

There was no other solution for her acute and potentially lethal blockage. Initially, she declined consent for the operation because she had read an article written by an alternative doctor who contended that bypass surgery was largely unnecessary. Obviously, he hadn't witnessed cardiology patients die of heart attacks in his parking lot as we have. Fortunately, Janet was persuaded to have the procedure. Afterward, she safely embarked on a program of natural remedies that accelerated her recovery and improved her arterial, heart, and overall health.

Rates of complications from coronary artery bypass surgeries—such as heart attack, infection, stroke, and central nervous system dysfunction—are disturbing. People are naturally looking for less risky alternatives. However, bypass is a sound approach to improve quality of life and possibly advance longevity when other alternative or conventional medical therapies fail to correct persistent chest pain and shortness of breath caused by coronary artery blockage.

The two sides of the coin—conventional therapy alone or alternative therapy alone—represent misguided medicine. Health professionals entrenched solely in one camp do their patients a major disservice. Smart medicine doesn't choose sides.

Sobering Numbers

The American Heart Association estimates that in 2002 approximately 70 million Americans had one or more forms of cardiovascular disease (CVD). In that year, CVD took 927,448 lives in the United States—that is, 1 out of every 2.6 deaths.

Coronary artery disease (CAD) alone accounted for 494,382 deaths, the single leading cause of death in the United States and the industrialized world. CAD develops when the coronary arteries supplying blood to the heart muscle narrow due to plaque buildup. About 335,000 people a year die of sudden cardiac arrest in hospital emergency rooms or before they ever receive medical attention.

Think Inflammation, Not Cholesterol

Cardiovascular disease (CVD) can kill in an instant by heart attack or stroke. Fifty percent of the time, the very first symptom is cardiac arrest.

Without warning, half of all people who have the disease die without ever knowing they had it.

CVD can also silently and slowly strangle the vitality of the most important muscle in your body—the heart muscle—which pumps life-sustaining blood and nutrients through the sixty thousand miles of blood vessels. The lining of those blood vessels becomes inflamed and can even be destroyed. Blockages develop and blood can't flow.

Medical science has come a long way in its understanding of what causes these scenarios. The pieces of the cardiovascular puzzle are coming together and new information is shoving aside cholesterol as the dreaded boogeyman of cardiovascular disease. If cholesterol were the omnikiller, then everyone with heart disease would have high cholesterol. Yet half of all heart attacks occur in individuals with normal cholesterol.

Recently, a radical shift has swept through cardiology. Inflammation has been identified as the most important factor in the formation of plaque and arterial disease. Along with this breakthrough have come new tools with which to precisely diagnose risk, identify specific inflammatory markers, and effectively treat both stable and unstable arterial disease.

The truth is that the body sustains a daily toxic assault and forms plaque as a result. We predict that *plaque reversal* will become the new buzzwords. In New Cardiology, we feel it is more important for you to know if your blood is toxic, the state of your dental health, how much insulin your diet produces, and how you handle stress.

We may prescribe a cholesterol-lowering drug but not for the reason you think. We may recommend it because it also beats down arterial inflammation. At the same time, we may want you to start on a simple supplement regimen of fish oil, magnesium, CoQ10, niacin, vitamin C, and nattokinase, which can offer you more lifesaving benefits than many medical drugs without side effects.

In New Cardiology, we check cholesterol, but we are more concerned about homocysteine, a troublesome substance that builds up in the body if you're short of certain vitamins, creating inflammation and sticky blood. We want to check substances called Lp(a), fibrinogen, ferritin, and C-reactive protein (CRP). We want to determine the calcium score in your coronary arteries—a new measurement that predicts heart attack risk better than traditional tests.

You may not have heard about these things before. But they are very central to understanding how inflammation and plaque clog and consume arteries, consequently destroying heart function. We will tell you how you can extinguish the silent fire of inflammation, stop the destructive clogging of your arteries, and reduce your risk of heart disease, stroke, and sudden cardiac death.

You can do so much for yourself, whether you have acute or chronic disease or just want to prevent CVD from developing. Many natural methods work superbly, even if you have a family history of serious heart disease. But there are also times when patients must resort to medication and perhaps even surgery. In those cases, lifestyle and nutritional supplements can make all the difference in recovery and long-term prognosis.

Here are some of the major points we'll be covering in the pages ahead:

- How to tell if you are at risk for CVD and why it's harder to tell in women

- How killer inflammation and plaque develop in your body, often silently

- The obsession with cholesterol and why we need to change our focus

- The most important causes of inflammation and plaque, including the smallest known bacteria in the world, the overconsumption of sweets, and the bad fat contained in 75 percent of processed foods

- Sophisticated new testing procedures that offer great lifesaving potential and hopefully will soon become part of a standard approach to prevention

- Medical drugs—their upsides and downsides

- Nutritional supplements that block inflammation, stabilize and perhaps even reverse plaque, and some that actually "eat" clots

- The amazing power of CoQ10, L-carnitine, and D-ribose—three super supplements that keep your heart pumping at the max

- Getting the lead out, along with mercury and other toxic substances that poison your blood and arteries

- An absolutely artery-friendly diet

- Exercise and a big secret that gets habitual exercise shirkers moving as well as people who don't have the energy to exercise

- Attitudes and lifestyle

- Our detailed how-to program with suggestions for healing, prevention, and improving abnormal test results

Are You at Risk?

In the summer of 2004, former president Bill Clinton underwent quadruple coronary artery bypass surgery after experiencing chest pains and shortness of breath. In bypass surgery, also called open heart surgery, doctors remove one or more vessels from the chest, arm, leg, or stomach and attach them to arteries carrying blood to the heart, thus detouring blood around blockages.

Clinton thought his blockage was probably caused in part by genetics. His mother's family has a history of heart disease. But he also admitted the possibility of self-inflicted damage during "those years when I was too careless about what I ate." As president, he was known for his fast-food habit.

Clinton's case underscores the importance of listening to your body. The ex-president hadn't been feeling well, yet his doctors said all was well when they first checked him out. But he insisted that something was wrong and followed his intuition. Further tests showed that Clinton indeed had acute coronary artery disease (CAD), meaning severe blockage of the coronary arteries that feed the heart. He could have dropped dead at any minute. He chose to have bypass surgery.

Classic Cardiac Symptoms

These symptoms are not 100 percent gender-specific. Women generally experience more vaguely defined symptoms than men.

Men
- Midchest pressure
- Shortness of breath
- Dull pain between the shoulder blades
- Achiness in the jaw
- Pain in the left arm or elbow
- Profuse sweating

Women
- Acute breathlessness
- Sudden, profound fatigue
- Dull, aching chest discomfort (vague)
- Jaw or neck pain
- Pain in the left arm or elbow
- Abdominal discomfort, nausea, vomiting
- Dizziness, even blackouts

The biggest reason that people die of CAD is they deny what their bodies are telling them. Clinton listened to his symptoms. He had chest pain. Shortness of breath. Something was wrong. He went back to the hospital. An angiogram revealed the high-grade blockages. His situation was life-threatening and required aggressive treatment. He was handled very well by conventional medicine.

Often, there is no such happy ending. You probably know somebody who died in his forties from a heart attack without any warning. Keep in mind that 90 percent of coronary disease is asymptomatic—a silent process eroding the arteries. In half those cases, sudden death is the very first symptom. Those with symptoms are lucky because they can be evaluated like President Clinton.

Usually, Americans seek medical attention regarding cardiac risk only when lab tests show their cholesterol, triglycerides, or blood sugar to be high. These tests have been done routinely for decades because of the famous Framingham Heart Study, an ambitious health research project organized by the National Heart, Lung, and Blood Institute in 1948 to uncover the general causes of heart disease and stroke. CVD was largely undiagnosed before 1920, but in the ensuing years became a public health concern as the death rates from heart attacks rose steeply and reached epidemic proportions.

The Framingham project sought to identify common factors or characteristics contributing to CVD based on long-term monitoring of a large group of participants who had not yet developed overt symptoms of disease or suffered a heart attack or a stroke. Over time, the Framingham research singled out age, family history of CVD, blood cholesterol, blood pressure, cigarette smoking, and diabetes. The research said that the more risk factors you have, the more you are at risk for heart attack. For example, if you have high blood pressure, high cholesterol, high triglycerides, and are a smoker, you stand a higher risk to develop a cardiac event than if you had just one or two factors.

A cardiac event refers to a blockage of life-sustaining blood and oxygen in an artery leading to the heart. Even though we are cardiologists, we are also concerned about the arteries to the brain. The similarity between a heart attack and a stroke is this: both events are caused by arterial blockages or plaque rupture in a vital vessel. Usually a clot (thrombus) or a piece of plaque from somewhere in the body or in the immediate artery breaks off, lodging at a point where it cannot pass through. The blockage then cuts off the circulation, leading to oxygen deprivation of the tissue that the artery serves. The brain or the heart infarct, meaning that downstream tissue dies from lack of nourishing oxygen.

In the heart, clots are more likely to occur in areas already partially blocked or where there is existing vulnerable plaque. A piece of plaque could break off from the aorta or a carotid vessel and travel to the brain, or a piece of plaque could break off in a vessel in the brain itself, leading to occlusion of a vessel. One difference in the brain is that some strokes are hemorrhagic in nature, meaning they result from a ruptured blood vessel. The local hemorrhage causes tissue damage. High blood pressure is the primary cause of hemorrhagic stroke.

When a heart attack occurs, the heart muscle—the pump—has been affected. In a stroke, the occlusion or a bleed occurs in the brain circulation and the affected tissue in the brain. Both can and usually do occur abruptly.

Angina (chest pain) is a warning sign of disturbed circulation in the heart and is transient. No damage is done, but it must be evaluated. In the brain, a transient ischemic attack, or TIA, is a temporary disruption in blood flow, and it, too, should be taken seriously in a medical workup.

Traditional Signs and Symptoms of a Stroke

- Arm and leg weakness on the same side
- Weakness in facial muscles: may progress to one-sided facial droop
- Sudden headache
- Staggering gait; leg weakness or instability
- Imbalance; stumbling; difficulty walking or picking up objects
- Difficulty speaking (aphasia) and slurred speech
- Double vision or loss of vision in visual field on same side for both eyes

If arteries are blocked in the legs, walking is impaired. Cramping pain and weakness develops in the calves. This condition is called intermittent claudication.

Cardiologists have learned that when plaque buildup and blockage occur in arteries in one part of the body, such as the arteries to the heart or to the brain, there is usually blockage elsewhere. Translation: systemic disease.

Conventional cardiology treatments are typically brought into play when a person has major narrowing of an artery to the heart or the brain. New Cardiology can be implemented for a mere 10 percent narrowing. We think people should get a full range of important tests—the standard tests and the new ones—before symptoms ever arise. We want to work with people at an early date instead of waiting until they need a bypass or multiple medications that will cause side effects. But even if we get patients with advanced blockage, we are still able to use many of the same New Cardiology techniques.

In New Cardiology, doctors turn over more stones than just cholesterol and the standard Framingham risk factors. Framingham remains an honored model, but we go far beyond. This is because for years we have seen arteries full of plaque in nonsmokers with normal cholesterol and normal blood pressure.

Gender-Specific Issues

Man or woman, should you experience traditional or nontraditional symptoms of a heart attack or a stroke, call your physician immediately or get to an emergency care facility. In case of severe symptoms such as chest pain, fluctuations of consciousness, slurred speech, or profound sudden weakness on one side of the body, call 911.

Men

If you are a man in your thirties or forties and you develop erectile dysfunction (ED), it could be a sign of impaired blood flow to the penis and possible heart trouble in the not-too-distant future. There is a strong link between the two if the erectile problem isn't related to a psychological issue. Very often, young men will feign concern for their heart, asking their doctor for a Viagra prescription. Interestingly, Viagra was developed to treat angina. But men younger than fifty shouldn't have erectile dysfunction. Those who do are at increased risk of developing premature coronary artery disease. ED is angina of the reproductive organs.

Women

Three decades ago, the ratio of people admitted to coronary care units was roughly nine men to every woman. Unfortunately, this was not

The New Cardiology Risk Assessment

Here's a short and simple checklist that can determine your risk of a cardio-vascular event based on the New Cardiology approach. You'll need to get blood work and an electron beam tomography (EBT) scan. But the time spent will be worth your while because you'll get a good picture of your vulnerability. After you receive your test results, check the boxes that apply to you:

- ☐ A family history of cardiovascular events (heart attack, stroke) under the age of fifty.

- ☐ You are a male, or a "vitally exhausted" (meaning chronically fatigued, stressed-out) female

- ☐ An HDL (high-density lipoprotein) cholesterol level lower than 35 mg/dl (men) or 40 mg/dl (women)

- ☐ Triglycerides* higher than 150 ml/dl

- ☐ Triglyceride/HDL ratio higher than 4 to 1

- ☐ Homocysteine higher than 10 µmol/L

- ☐ Lp(a) higher than 30 mg/dl

- ☐ CRP (C-reactive protein) higher than 1.5 mg/L

- ☐ Fibrinogen higher than 350 mg/dl

- ☐ Fasting insulin above 17 microunits/L

- ☐ Resting blood pressure above 140/90

- ☐ EBT (scan for calcified plaque) score above 200

Each checkmark means 1 point. Add your points to get your total score. This informal test is not based on any official or medical association criteria but on our combined clinical experience. We would interpret your results as follows:

0–1   Minimum risk

2–3   Low risk

---

*Triglycerides are the chemical form of most fats in the body. Triglycerides in the blood come from dietary fats or from other calorie sources such as carbohydrates. Dietary calories not used immediately by tissues for energy are converted to triglycerides and stored in fat cells. Stored triglycerides are released as needed to meet energy demands. Excess triglycerides are linked to coronary artery disease in some people.

4–5   Moderate risk

6   Moderate to severe risk

over 7 Severe risk

You'll notice we have left off total cholesterol. As we will explain in the coming pages, there are other factors that we believe are more important.

Notice that we also left out smoking. That's because we assume you don't smoke. If you do, add 3 points. Smoking is a killer by anybody's standards.

---

because women required less treatment but because they received less treatment. In the past, women's pain was often written off by physicians as anxiety or as having a psychological cause. Frequently, a woman with chest symptoms or shortness of breath was sent home with a prescription for Valium or an antidepressant.

Even today, when a woman sees her doctor for symptom assessment, she may find herself caught up in a diagnostic dilemma. Because her symptoms are often less definitive or dramatic than those of men, her doctor may underestimate them or fail to order follow-up tests.

When a man over forty with arm or chest pain enters the ER, there's a good chance he'll be admitted to the hospital. But CVD symptoms in women might include discomfort in the chest that mimics indigestion—that feeling that if you could just burp you would feel more comfortable. Or it might be pain in the neck that radiates into the jaw or profound fatigue. Many women will write off their symptoms as the flu and not even seek medical attention. Cardiologists call these confounding cardiac signs atypical, meaning they don't fit the textbook scenario.

Even after many years as cardiologists and being aware of the unusual symptoms displayed by many women, we still find that CAD in women can be confusing. New research also suggests that women may more often experience nonclassic symptoms of a stroke than men.

Since symptoms can frequently be different and not the textbook presentation we quickly diagnose and treat in men, we encourage women to tune in to their intuition when they realize something is wrong. Act immediately. Avoid denial and don't rationalize symptoms. Remember that the leading cause of death and disability in women is heart disease and stroke.

You and Your Doctor

We are both information hounds. We regularly attend medical conferences and talk to researchers and clinicians in the fields of cardiology,
nutrition, and environmental medicine. Much of our clinical work is
innovative and, in a sense, five or ten years ahead of standard care. So,
many doctors may not feel comfortable with some of the ideas we discuss
in this book.

Our methods, however, are based on solid science that we have validated with countless patients. We often work with patients being seen by
other cardiologists and coordinate our efforts. We give these patients
additional options and a better chance to heal, with methods that may be
unfamiliar to their doctors.

The worst-case scenario would be no improvement with the nutritional supplements and other methods we recommend. But in our clinical experience, we usually see significant improvement when patients
follow the New Cardiology suggestions.

Cardiologists often see restenosis (renarrowing of the artery) after
an initial angioplasty. Many doctors will do another angioplasty. But in
New Cardiology we want to know why the artery narrowed and then
address the underlying cause. We may not be able to take away the
plaque, but we can take away the vulnerability. The patient may stabilize
and do great.

If you have been sick for years, be patient. This approach can get
you feeling better within a matter of months, sometimes within weeks.
Don't give up if you don't feel dramatically better overnight. Our recommendations don't generate quick, temporary fixes. They generate a lasting fix that arrests deterioration that would otherwise continue. Your

Do Not Discontinue Any Medication
Unless Your Doctor Says So

If you take prescription medication for your condition under a doctor's care,
please do not discontinue or alter your program without checking with your
physician. For your own protection, ask your doctor about any of the information you read here.

physiology—the way your body functions—indicates your future. And our approach influences physiology in a positive way. Your anatomy determines your present. We can't change your present, but we can influence your future.

Your doctor takes care of many other patients like you and may not have the time to study the new and complementary methods we discuss. Show your doctor this book. Hopefully, he or she may be interested in learning more about some of the ideas presented here.

PART ONE

How We Get Clogged

Chapter 1

Death by Inflammation

Inflammation is our body's first line of defense against injury or infection. It's what causes a burn to turn red or a bruise to swell. It's nature's design to help us heal. But if inflammation becomes chronic and goes into constant overdrive, it can cause disease.

In 2000, doctors at Harvard University published the first of a series of landmark research studies revealing the central role of inflammation in cardiovascular disease (CVD). Evidence from the Women's Health Study, a project that monitored the status of twenty-eight thousand initially healthy postmenopausal women, put a new risk factor into the spotlight: C-reactive protein (CRP), a key biochemical substance indicating the presence of vascular inflammation. People with the highest level of CRP had five times the risk of developing CVD and four times the risk of a heart attack or a stroke compared to individuals with the lowest level. CRP predicted risk in women who had none of the standard risk factors and was the best predictor among twelve risk factors studied, including cholesterol. The cardiologist Paul Ridker, who led the study, said that "we have to think of heart disease as an inflammatory disease, just as we think of rheumatoid arthritis as an inflammatory disease."

Ridker estimates that approximately 25 percent of Americans have a normal to low cholesterol level, lulling them into complacency, but at the same time they have an elevated CRP without knowing it. Millions of

Americans are unaware that they have an increased risk for future CVD, heart attack, or stroke.

Ridker's research confirmed what we as clinicians had suspected for years: that low-grade inflammation, like a silent, creeping fire, consumes arterial tissue and causes CVD. It leads to the weakening and eventual rupture of arterial plaques that directly trigger heart attacks and strokes. The CRP–inflammation link helps explain why more than half of heart attack and stroke victims have normal cholesterol levels.

Medical research has introduced us to other far-reaching and complex risk factors that go beyond the solitary threat of high cholesterol. Indeed, we have moved so far forward in recent years that the familiar model of diseased arteries as a network of inanimate pipes clogged by cholesterol-laden plaque seems almost as outmoded as the typewriter.

Life-threatening plaque is now regarded as an inflammatory injury—a lesion—that develops, almost like a boil, along the inner surface of the arterial walls where vital biological functions take place as blood rushes by. The walls become damaged by the inflammation—a process influenced by lifestyle, environment, and genetics. In some cases, the process unfolds slowly, stifling arterial wall chemistry and causing vessels to narrow. In other cases, deterioration occurs surprisingly fast, leading to vessel closure, stroke, or sudden death.

Plaque can be of two types. Stable plaque, covered with a fibrous cap, slowly expands inward and shrinks the diameter of blood vessels. Of greater danger is the vulnerable, unstable plaque, which can rupture and spill its noxious contents into the arteries and shut off blood flow. Identifying and combating the latter type of plaque has become the number one priority of today's cutting-edge cardiologists.

Indicative of a turnaround in thinking about the causes of CVD, the American Heart Association and the Centers for Disease Control and Prevention published new recommendations for CVD screening in 2003 that included a test for CRP. Today you may see posters on laboratory walls with information for patients about this new and potentially life-saving blood test. There is more to inflammation than CRP and more to CVD than inflammation, but we see this kind of public awareness effort as a good first step in getting out the message about inflammation and CVD.

Cardiovascular System 101

The heart and its network of blood vessels deliver oxygen and metabolic fuel to the cells. Think of your heart as a fist-sized, cone-shaped muscular

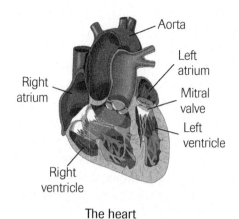

Aorta

Left atrium

Right atrium

Mitral valve

Left ventricle

Right ventricle

The heart

pump wrapped around four chambers. The chambers are connected by a series of one-way valves that let blood flow in one side and out the other. Oxygen-poor "used" blood returning to the heart collects in the right atrium chamber and is funneled into the right ventricle, which pumps it into the lungs to pick up oxygen. Oxygenated blood returns to the left atrium, passes through the mitral valve into the left ventricle, and is pumped out with great force (in a healthy heart) into the main artery of the body, the aorta. From the aorta, other arteries branch off to feed the body, including the two coronary arteries that supply the heart muscle.

Blood moves through your body's sixty thousand miles of blood vessels known as the circulatory system. Think of this system as the branches of a tree with many offshoots or a river with many tributaries. Large arteries branch off into smaller arterioles. These, in turn, branch off into the smallest vessels, called capillaries, which feed the cells of the body, then carry wastes and deoxygenated blood back out into venules (small veins), then into larger veins, and finally back to the right atrium.

This elaborate system needs to be clear to accommodate the forceful contractions of the heart and permit strong blood flow. The walls of the blood vessels have to be smooth and free of obstruction. We will concentrate on the arteries, since CVD primarily affects arteries rather than veins.

As Goes the Endothelium, So Go You

Artery walls are not hard and firm. Instead, they are composed of smooth muscle that contracts and expands in metronomic response to the rhythm of the heart, accommodating the pulsatile flow of blood. They are a living, breathing, dynamic organ, not a static system of tubes and pipes.

We are most concerned with the innermost layer of the wall known as the endothelium. The blood meets the vessel walls at the endothelium. Though only one cell thick, this permeable lining carries out critical

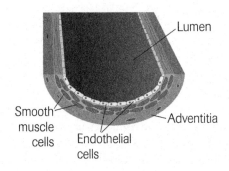

The endothelial lining

molecular exchanges between the blood-borne contents floating through the lumen and the smooth muscle and adventitial tissues behind it that form the bulk and structure of the arteries. A healthy endothelium produces chemical substances that allow for the normal expansion and relaxation of blood vessels. Endothelial health is critical to cardiovascular health. If you have a 40 to 50 percent narrowing of the arteries and impaired endothelial function, you are at greater risk for an adverse event than if you had an 80 percent narrowing of the arteries with intact endothelial function.

The endothelial lining is extremely delicate and sensitive to injury. It can be damaged by a variety of insults. Of course, you can injure the endothelium, along with the entire artery wall, if you cut yourself and slice an artery. Trauma aside, we are concerned with the steady damage from inflammation that develops over time from a less than healthy lifestyle. Unhealthy habits include overeating refined, packaged, and processed foods with lots of sugar, unnatural fats, and chemical preservatives; not eating enough fresh fruits and vegetables and not drinking enough water; smoking; and not being physically active. Living in an environment where you are regularly exposed to pollution and contaminants is an inflammation risk factor. Stress associated with work, relationships, and financial pressures can compound the problem.

Silent Inflammation Starts Early

A middle-aged person may go to the doctor, perhaps complaining of shortness of breath or maybe just for a checkup, and hear that his cholesterol is too high and he has the beginnings of atherosclerosis, commonly known as hardening of the arteries.

The news comes with a loud jolt. But the process itself has been going on silently for a long time, starting at a surprisingly young age. Studies going back to Korean War and Vietnam War casualties show that even some teenagers have early arterial disease. More recently, researchers specializing in the study of early-onset atherosclerosis reported in the medical journal *Circulation* that 20 to 25 percent of young people (aged fourteen to thirty-five) autopsied after death from homicide, auto accident, or suicide already had a major lesion in the coronary arteries. The study was performed on three thousand bodies.

- Just over 3 percent of men aged fifteen to nineteen had 40 percent narrowing or greater in at least one coronary vessel. The prevalence increased to nearly 20 percent in thirty- to thirty-four-year-old men.

- Narrowing of 40 percent or more was not found in women before the age of twenty-five. Occlusions of this magnitude were found in 8 percent of those aged thirty to thirty-four.

- The presence of risk factors (such as smoking and diabetes) increased the likelihood of significant narrowing.

These numbers show that millions already have significant coronary disease at an early age. Most likely, they don't know it.

The message from these statistics is clear: you should not wait to begin a preventive program. Start as early as possible.

Arterial Hot Spots

The major cardiac hot spots are the left main coronary artery—the "left main" for short—and locations just beyond where it splits into the left anterior descending and left circumflex arteries on the outer surface of the heart. These blood vessels supply the front and side walls of the heart muscle.

The higher up in these vessels that blockages develop, the more damage that occurs "downstream." The left anterior descending artery is the potential site of the most dangerous lesion. We call it the "widow maker." It puts two-thirds of the heart muscle in jeopardy. The

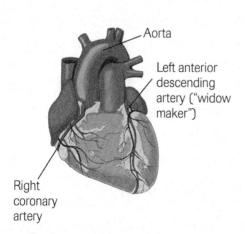

The heart and coronary hot spots

Aorta

Left anterior descending artery ("widow maker")

Right coronary artery

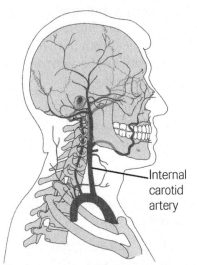

The internal carotid arteries, the most important vessels feeding the brain

right coronary artery feeds the bottom and back portions of the heart muscle.

A blockage compromises the supply of oxygen and other blood-borne nutrients to the cells served by the artery and its branches. Denied their essential raw materials, these cells fail to generate adequate energy to sustain themselves and their multiple functions. If the blockage is incomplete, the cells starve. Pumping function ceases, but the cells remain alive. If the blockage closes the vessel, the cells die, and a myocardial infarct—a heart attack—is the result.

In the neck, the carotid arteries are the hot spots because they feed the front of the brain where you do your thinking. A stroke is like having a heart attack in the brain. There are four major arteries going into the brain: the left and right carotid arteries, which split into the external and internal branches; and the left and right vertebral arteries, which split into vessels serving the back of the brain. If a major blood vessel becomes blocked (especially before the split), a stroke is likely.

If you could take a miniature close-up camera and position it at a site of arterial inflammation, you would see a bulge along the artery wall, making the lumen (the flow area) narrower and less easily passable. The endothelium would look stretched out, like overstressed elastic. The spaces between the endothelial cells would be larger. Under the cap of this endothelial bulge, the plaque lesion forms—a virtual witch's brew of toxicity.

Narrowed arteries place a strain on the cardiovascular system and create all sorts of other health problems, as the heart is overstressed to pump harder and compensate for the partially obstructed blood flow. In turn, this raises blood pressure, leading to further cardiac strain.

The Role of the Immune System

The immune system protects the body from foreign invaders such as bacteria. It fields a variety of cells armed with different weapons to fight the enemy. Some of these cells are released by the immune system and others by the injured tissue itself. Some are designed to engulf invading organisms, others to gobble them up, others to cart off the debris, and still others to seal off the injury and allow healing to begin.

This internal defense force is constantly challenged as it is involved in battle and repair operations. Without such a robust system, you would be overwhelmed by every germ you encounter and every injury you sustain.

Inflammation takes place when immune cells are summoned to the site of an injury such as an insect bite, a laceration, gum disease, or a broken ankle. The composition of cells depends on the nature and the location of the challenge, but all cause some characteristics of inflammation, namely redness, heat, and sometimes swelling. In the case of a viral or bacterial assault, the system may respond with fever, diarrhea, or nausea in addition to any localized distress.

In any case, the inflammatory response stirs up a complex array of chemicals throughout the body. In this alert mode, a normal defensive reaction in one place can contribute to unwanted inflammation elsewhere. An infection in the gums can leak bacteria into the bloodstream. The bacteria may find fertile ground in a weakened arterial wall or a defective heart valve and fan the flames of inflammation there. In rheumatoid arthritis, a highly inflammatory condition, researchers have discovered that a woman's risk for heart attack is doubled.

Inflammation may or may not be obvious. It can take place on a subtle or silent level. From head to toe, your body is always in a process of repairing itself, with countless mini-inflammation dramas going on that you are not aware of as you go about your daily business or sleep. Inflammation in the arteries is an example of this below-the-radar-screen activity.

From Inflammation to Plaque

The delicate endothelium can become damaged from a variety of elements, including cigarette smoke, toxic chemicals and metals, bad fats, poor diet, elevated insulin, bacteria, high blood pressure, and excess stress.

Singly, or in combination, these elements kindle inflammation that can evolve into plaque. Following is a stage-by-stage description of the process.

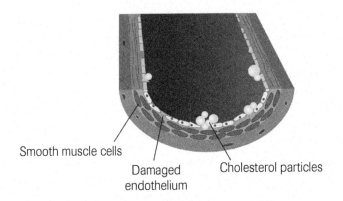

Smooth muscle cells

Damaged
endothelium

Cholesterol particles

The start of arterial damage

Stage 1

Under siege, the normally smooth endothelium becomes permeable or porous, attracting fatty particles such as circulating cholesterol. These particles wriggle into the lining and disturb biological activities. Usually, though not always, this occurs at locations where the endothelium tends to be under extra pressure. A typical hot spot is where the left main coronary artery splits into the anterior descending and circumflex arteries.

Once cholesterol becomes wedged in the arterial wall, a chemical process may take place in which the fatty molecules are damaged by free radicals to form oxidized LDL (low-density lipoprotein) cholesterol. Soon the ever-vigilant immune system takes notice that something is amiss and needs attention. The system goes into action.

Stage 2

Local cells surrounding a distressed site release immune chemicals that initiate an inflammatory process. The intima, the layer of tissue just behind the endothelium, secretes adhesion molecules to create a sticky endothelial surface like fly paper. Blood cells adhere, including mono-cytes, circulating immune cells instrumental in the inflammatory response. Meanwhile, the besieged endothelium secretes endothelin and other distress-signaling agents.

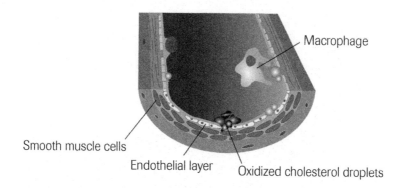

The inflammatory damage intensifies

Stage 3

The endothelium and intima now release other chemicals. They cause more circulating monocytes to swarm across the endothelial barrier and mature into full-fledged scavengers called macrophages that are designed to seek and destroy foreign objects. Under ordinary circumstances, macrophages engulf invading cells, consume them, and are eliminated from the body by other specialized immune cells. But the developing situation here is no longer ordinary.

Stage 4

Oxidized LDL is not benign. It is toxic to the macrophage. Oxidized LDL immobilizes the macrophage, preventing it from returning to the bloodstream. The stressed macrophage sends out an SOS—a proinflammatory distress signal that draws other white cells into the area, where they, too, are destroyed by the oxidized LDL. Under the microscope, we see a fatty streak made up of dying macrophages loaded with oxidized LDL layering out from the inner area of the artery wall.

Stage 5

Proinflammatory substances gather in a seething commune of cytokines, enzymes (proteins responsible for stimulating other chemical reactions in

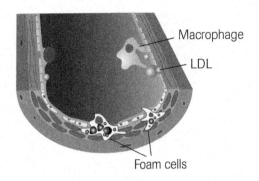

The lesion grows . . .

the body), and growth factors. They go by such names as interleukin-1 (IL-1), tumor necrosis factor-alpha (TNF-alpha), interleukin-6 (IL-6), macrophage colony-stimulating factor, and various interferons. These chemicals increase the stickiness of the endothelial wall and make it even more permeable to white blood cells and LDL cholesterol, which continue to enter and burrow inside. The lesion grows and attracts other chemical bedfellows such as CRP and fibrinogen, all produced in the liver and dispatched to sites of injury or infection.

C-reactive protein is probably the most pervasive of these substances, abundantly present in all inflammatory fluids, in the intimal layer of the atherosclerotic artery, and in the foam cells (LDL-engorged macrophages) within the lesions of the forming plaque. CRP stimulates cells to release tissue factor, a protein central to the clotting process.

Remember that the body wants to heal or seal off any injury. That's the purpose of these individual chemicals. But nature's plan backfires. The lesion becomes stickier and keeps attracting dangerous chemicals as it grows—a truly vicious cycle. Bacteria and toxic metals join in.

Think of plaque progression in terms of the body responding to a growing internal infection. The immune system's natural reactions feed on itself, creating a general state of inflammatory alert.

Stage 6

The body now calls in yet another set of chemicals designed to create a hard seal over the roiling inflammation. They team up with white blood cells, collagen and elastin (two important proteins that make up connective tissue), and platelets to form a tough, fibrous cap.

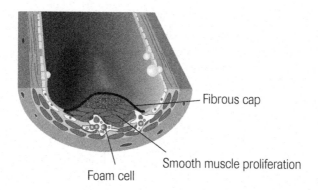

Fibrous cap

Smooth muscle proliferation

Foam cell

. . . into a potentially dangerous plaque

Under the cap, dead cells pile up and decay. Pus develops. This necrotic core becomes a growing plaque. It's like a boil within the artery wall.

Typically, this drama is not confined to a single location but unfolds at various points along arterial walls throughout the system. Inflammatory mediators released at one vulnerable site can agitate endothelial cells elsewhere, converting stable plaque into vulnerable plaque. Vulnerability and the tendency for plaque rupture increases. Plaque begets plaque. If you have it in your heart arteries, you most likely have it in your carotids and aorta. And elsewhere.

At some advanced point in the inflammatory process, calcium becomes deposited in the struggling arterial cells as part of their effort to produce adequate energy. When they open to calcium, the cells also let in

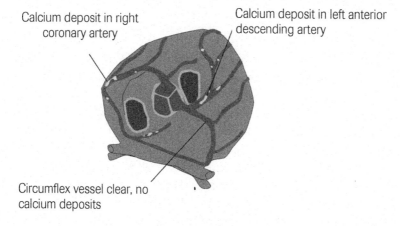

Calcium deposit in right coronary artery

Calcium deposit in left anterior descending artery

Circumflex vessel clear, no calcium deposits

An example of plaque in the coronary arteries

circulating toxic metals such as lead and cadmium. This is not a clearly understood phenomenon. All we know is that calcium is there—and shouldn't be—making up about a fifth of the volume of the plaque and contributing to its hardness.

Stage 7

The affected arteries reshape themselves to accommodate plaque buildup. As the lesions grow, the arterial wall expands and bulges to accommodate them. This process is called remodeling. Lesions soon begin to obstruct the lumen through which blood is flowing and the arterial walls begin losing elasticity.

Stage 8

At this point, significant plaque deposits exist in various stages, and further developments determine whether a heart attack or a stroke follow. Subsequent events can take two possible scenarios.

Scenario 1: Stable Plaque

In this scenario, the fibrous cap holds firm, withstanding the roiling changes from within and the immune system's siege from outside. There could be a number of reasons for this resiliency under duress:

- Changes in lifestyle that reduce the toxins entering the body—for instance, eating less bad fats and quitting smoking
- Beginning a treatment program designed to quell inflammation and repair the endothelial layer
- A genetic predisposition to a lower-level inflammatory response

Hardened, constricted arteries cause the heart to work harder to pump blood through narrower blood vessels. This can lead to angina—chest pains commonly associated with heart disease.

Stable plaque can cause symptoms if the heart weakens due to chronic oxygen deficiency or if the artery is so narrow that it becomes completely blocked. Surprisingly, this dynamic is responsible for relatively few heart attacks. Many people with plaque-ridden arteries live well into their eighties and nineties—as long as the plaque is stable. Often, with slowly closing arteries, the body forms natural bypasses.

Heart failure occurs if the heart cannot pump sufficient amounts of blood to the rest of the body. Fluid accumulates in the lungs, ankles, or legs, creating general fatigue and shortness of breath. If leg arteries are affected, numbness, fatigue, or pain may be experienced in the lower extremities, especially upon walking. This situation is called intermittent claudication, a prime symptom of peripheral artery disease.

Scenario 2: Vulnerable (Unstable) Plaque

This scenario carries the most danger. The fibrous cap starts to erode as a result of ongoing inflammatory assault from within the lesion and from outside. In the necrotic core, cellular breakdown and release of inflammatory substances create internal destabilization. Foam cells, for instance, release chemicals that can weaken the protective cap.

New plaque zones form externally, and the inflammatory chemicals they release, together with circulating destructive substances such as free radicals, also lead to destabilization. A leak develops and macrophages enter. They produce enzymes and inflammatory substances, along with clotting factors such as fibrinogen, to reseal the injury. However, the lesion swells and the fibrous cap continues to degrade until suddenly the cap ruptures.

The noxious contents spill into the bloodstream. Platelets and clotting agents converge to plug the leak. A thrombus (blood clot) forms immediately. The clot can obstruct a vessel on the spot, or if it is small enough, can flow downstream until it clogs a smaller vessel. Or a piece of the plaque cap can break off and do the same.

Inflammation causes the plaque to rupture, and the rupture is what kills most of the time. We used to call this event coronary thrombosis. Now we call it plaque rupture. Vulnerable, oxidized, inflamed plaques will rupture. Plaque rupture can lead to three potentially devastating events: acute heart attack, death from arrhythmia (the heart stops or races wildly because of electrical instability due to the sudden loss of oxygen), and, if it occurs in the carotid arteries or the brain, a stroke.

In emergency rooms and coronary care units, we apply clot-busting medication to alleviate the clot component of arterial obstruction. Then we do bypass surgery or dilate the narrowing and place a stent. This saves lives and limits heart muscle damage.

The size of the lesion means far less than its stability. Today, medical science allows us to pinpoint these plaques and stabilize or even reverse them before an event occurs.

If an occluded blood vessel can be expanded by just a fraction, blood flow can be improved considerably. This is what we try to do with medication and, in New Cardiology, with combinations of medication and nutritional supplements. Getting the blood vessel to relax or just open up slightly—what we call plaque reversal—produces an incredible effect. A mere 10 percent increase in vessel diameter from, say, 90 percent narrowing to 80 percent, will double blood flow.

In the old cardiology, the focus was on percent of blockage of the artery. We did nothing until a 70 percent narrowing was seen on the angiogram, then we did angioplasty or bypass surgery. In New Cardiology, we focus on the integrity and function of the endothelium—that is, the biology of the cells lining the arteries. We never give up because of high-grade narrowing. And we don't hold off treating a patient just because only a moderate narrowing is seen. We know we can always influence the biology of the lining of the cells.

The Speed of Plaque

How fast does plaque develop into a killer? That depends.

We have been shocked many times by people who form plaques within six months. All cardiologists have seen this. That's the nature of coronary artery disease. It can be like a snowball rolling down the hill. It gathers bulk as it increases momentum.

Stress can speed things up. For a cardiac patient, emotional stress is deadly. Blood vessels can spasm and tighten up, creating more deficiency to the heart. There could also be some lesser plaque that our diagnostics don't pick up—for example, 10 or 20 percent blockage—or the plaque can develop inside the wall where it can't be seen.

Plaque is dynamic. Left to its own devices, it will increase in size. If it develops substantially but very slowly, the body's intelligence can form natural bypasses. We call these collaterals. A patient may have a slowly closing coronary artery and not have a heart attack. A narrowed artery does not always require surgery.

Chapter 2

The Cholesterol Obsession

Years ago, like most cardiologists, we pushed patients to undergo angiograms (invasive heart catheterizations), whether they had CVD symptoms or not, just because their cholesterol reached 300 or higher. We did this because our profession believed that high cholesterol was the *big* cause of heart disease. We sincerely believed all people with high cholesterol were in danger. We needed to see just how bad their arteries were.

Many times we found diseased arteries, but often the angiogram revealed normal arteries. No disease at all. At first it made no sense. We just *knew* that the disease was there. We were convinced that cholesterol caused heart disease. And when we did angiograms on people beyond middle age and saw normal arteries, we were shocked. We couldn't understand how a cholesterol level over 300 did nothing to some patients. This was the influence of the cholesterol paradigm, a misconception dominating cardiology thinking for decades.

We began asking the patients with high cholesterol but no signs of disease what they were doing. They would say they had been taking vitamins and antioxidants. We were conventional cardiologists getting lessons from our patients.

The ABCs of Cholesterol

Every new patient we see asks about lowering his or her cholesterol, sometimes before we even measure it. Patients assume that their level is too high, an assumption fed by decades of cholesterol bashing.

Contrary to cholesterol's negative reputation, you and your body cannot function without it. Cholesterol is a basic raw material that enzymes convert into vitamin D, steroid hormones (such as estrogen, progesterone, testosterone, and cortisol), and the bile acids needed for digestion. You need cholesterol to construct the semipermeable membrane that surrounds your cells. You also need it to regenerate damaged endothelial cells.

The liver produces this fatlike waxy substance—about 800 mg a day, enough to cover your body's needs. You may also get cholesterol in your diet if you eat meat, eggs, and dairy such as milk and cheese. If you eat these cholesterol-rich foods, your liver makes less. If you eat less cholesterol, your liver makes more.

Cholesterol, being a fatty substance, is not soluble in water or blood. So your liver coats it with a protein wrapper that permits it to enter your circulatory system. The protein acts like a passport, allowing cholesterol to travel throughout your system.

You've no doubt heard the term *lipoprotein* in connection with cholesterol. *Lipo* means "fat." So a lipoprotein contains molecules of cholesterol (fat) enveloped in protein. The liver makes and then dispatches these cholesterol–protein combinations into the bloodstream as water-soluble LDL cholesterol lipoprotein. Cells in need of cholesterol will display an LDL cholesterol receptor on their outer membrane. The circulating LDL lipoprotein stops at the cell, attaches to a receptor site on the membrane, and offloads its cholesterol cargo. Inside the cell, the cholesterol is used as needed. Cells not needing cholesterol don't display the cholesterol receptor and the circulating lipoprotein floats by without stopping.

No matter how high the blood cholesterol level, a healthy cell cannot be overfilled with cholesterol. The exception to the rule is cholesterol oxidized by omnipresent and destructive molecular fragments called free radicals. Like a gate crasher, oxidized cholesterol particles enter into cells in excessive numbers and cause cellular toxicity.

In this manner, oxidized cholesterol enters into already inflamed arterial tissue and contributes to atherosclerosis and plaque, as we described in the last chapter. Cholesterol itself is not the culprit. Nature didn't equip you with a system designed to kill you. The problem lies in an *inability to process cholesterol properly* and/or an *inability for the body's antioxidant system to guard against oxidation of cholesterol.*

Cholesterol present in the circulation beyond the body's needs or within a cell beyond the needs of that cell serves no useful purpose and can be oxidized by free radicals. Nature understands this threat well and endowed our bodies with a removal process known as reverse cholesterol transport that extracts excess cholesterol from cells and from the walls of blood vessels.

To make this happen, the body needs a substance called phosphatidylcholine (PC), obtained in the diet from foods like fish, eggs, wheat germ, brussels sprouts, and broccoli. Lecithin cholesterol acyl transferase (LCAT), an enzyme present in the circulation, removes a fatty acid particle from PC and attaches it to cholesterol. The resulting entity, called a cholesterol ester, is then "grabbed" by another type of circulating lipoprotein called HDL—the so-called good cholesterol. HDL transports the ester back to the liver. The liver turns it into a bile salt, a digestive enzyme that helps break down dietary fat in the small intestine. Afterward, this by-product descends into the colon to be excreted along with digestive wastes.

We've simplified the scenario, but the bottom line is that these conversions naturally lower the content of cholesterol in the blood. A lower concentration of blood cholesterol also serves to coax excess cholesterol out of cells, including the cells that line blood vessels, and into the circulation. Thus, the reverse cholesterol transport system helps keep arteries clear of disease by removing one of the inflammation–plaque conspirators. LCAT, the enzyme that converts cholesterol into an ester, is activated by PC but is poisoned by heavy metals such as lead, cadmium, and especially mercury.

The Who's Who of Cholesterol

Good cholesterol. Bad cholesterol. What's "good" and what's "bad"? And why? The following explanation should help put the members of the cholesterol family in perspective.

Good Cholesterol: HDL

High-density lipoprotein acts like a garbage truck, picking up the ester-converted oxidized LDL and bringing it back to the liver. HDL has a stable personality, moves easily through the bloodstream, and doesn't stick to the arterial wall.

Also Good Cholesterol: Nonoxidized LDL

Low-density lipoprotein has gotten a bad rap. This is your basic cholesterol (wrapped in protein) that contributes to the many cholesterol needs of your body, including the making of hormones and cell membranes.

Bad Cholesterol: Oxidized LDL

Good turns to bad when LDL becomes oxidized by free radicals. Unless transported away by HDL, it sticks to artery walls, forming foam cells, which in turn attract blood-clotting components such as fibrin, platelets, and white blood cells. The foam cells become proinflammatory, swelling up, multiplying, and accelerating the inflammation and plaque formation process.

The Good-Turned-Ugly Cholesterol: Lipoprotein(a)

This cholesterol comprises one LDL molecule chemically bound to an attachment protein called apolipoprotein(a). In a healthy body, Lp(a) circulates and carries out repair and restoration work on the structural integrity of damaged blood vessel walls. The protein component promotes blood clotting and inhibits your body's blood clot–dissolving system, nature's mechanism to prevent excessive blood loss from a damaged vessel. Lp(a) also promotes vessel wall cellular growth and proliferation, and its LDL cholesterol is incorporated into the regenerating cells. Essentially, Lp(a) functions as a beneficial repair molecule, an artery patch.

Some individuals can have too much Lp(a) because of genetics. The risk also rises dangerously in the presence of atherosclerosis and constant damage to arterial walls. Then Lp(a) goes from useful to ugly. The body produces more to meet the repair demand. Lp(a) concentrates at the sites of damage. It binds with two structural amino acids—lysine and proline—within the wall of a damaged or weakened blood vessel, dumps its LDL cargo, and promotes the deposition of circulating, oxidized LDL into the wall, thus contributing to the buildup of plaque.

Lp(a) also promotes the formation of blood clots on top of the forming plaque. This narrows the vessel and worsens symptoms. If the clots are large enough, they can occlude an artery. We now know that most heart attacks are due to a large clot developing in vessels with moderate narrowings. Therefore, with Lp(a) present, even 50 percent blockage can make this situation dangerous.

Low-Density/High-Density Cholesterol: What Does It Mean?

Twenty-five years ago, blood cholesterol was simply blood cholesterol. We didn't know about lipoproteins and "good" and "bad" cholesterol. The researcher who initially identified the HDL and LDL components did so by spinning blood plasma in a centrifuge. The subfractions separated out according to their density. The LDL particle, lower in density, floated to the top. The HDL particle sank to the bottom. Thus the names—which have nothing to do with their function in the body.

The Making of a Killer Reputation

Society's obsession with cholesterol goes back to the famous Framingham Heart Study initiated in 1948 and the research of Ancel Keys, a brilliant public health scientist at the University of Minnesota. It was Keys who developed the famous K-ration (named for him) of World War II, a lightweight but nutritionally compact military field ration.

The Framingham study looked at the diet, lifestyles, and environments of a large number of families and turned up a correlation between high cholesterol and heart attacks. It was around this time that Keys discovered and quantified a relationship between the fat composition of diet and serum cholesterol level.

Keys's group collected statistics worldwide relating to heart disease deaths and fat consumption. Although more than twenty countries had such data at the time, Keys applied the statistics from seven countries that supported the animal fat (cholesterol)–heart disease theory, namely Italy, Greece, the former Yugoslavia, the Netherlands, Finland, the United States, and Japan. Keys's famous Seven Countries Study came to a number of influential conclusions, including:

- Population death rates from coronary heart disease could be predicted by knowing the average serum cholesterol.

- A strong correlation existed between heart disease incidence and average saturated fat intake.

In 1956, the American Heart Association drew on the combined Framingham and Keys conclusions and declared that "the cause of coronary heart disease was butter, lard, beef, and eggs." The medical world thus settled into the "cholesterol is the cause of heart disease" paradigm. The U.S. government sponsored efforts to educate the public about lowering cholesterol as a means of reducing the risk of heart disease. Currently the "official" target level for total cholesterol is 200 mg/dl or less and 40 mg/dl or higher for HDL.

If you consider all the research and just look at cardiovascular mortality in men, the lower the cholesterol level the better. The higher the worse. But not in women. In women, cholesterol is less predictive of cardiac death. Moreover, when you look at all other causes of death, people with higher cholesterol have less cancer, respiratory failure, automobile accidents, and suicides.

Accidents and suicides? The connection: you need cholesterol to make brain cells. A level too low (around 160 mg/dl) has, in fact, been linked to depression, aggression, and cerebral hemorrhages. Low cholesterol can also promote global amnesia because proper nerve transmission is affected. You need cholesterol for memory.

Cholesterol helps neutralize toxins produced by bacteria that swarm into the bloodstream from the gut when the system is weak. So your body also uses cholesterol to fight infections. The total blood level goes up when you have an infection and HDL falls because it is being used up in the fight.

The balance sheet shows that cholesterol protects against all causes of illness outside of cardiovascular disease. But if you have heart failure and high cholesterol, you actually fare better than someone with a low cholesterol level.

No one educates the public about cholesterol's varied benefits and essential roles in the body. Years of blaming cholesterol as the bad boy of heart disease has distorted the image of a totally necessary ingredient for the body's normal functioning.

The Unmaking of a Killer Reputation

Cholesterol has been misrepresented and thus poorly understood. A gross misconception has grown out of a multitude of studies suggesting that cholesterol is the enemy. Take the Seven Countries Study, for instance. The lowest rate for cancer and heart disease of all the countries was

Greece, and more specifically, the Greek island of Crete, where not a single heart attack was registered among the half-million population during a ten-year period.

The average citizen of Crete, according to the study, had a cholesterol level well above 200, perhaps because of all the goat cheese and full-fat yogurt consumed. Obviously, high saturated fat and cholesterol intake here didn't translate into higher levels of heart disease—just the opposite, in fact.

Turning to France, epidemiological data show that despite a rich, high-cholesterol diet—and an average cholesterol level well over 200—the French have one of the lowest incidences of heart disease in the developed world. Though red wine was initially thought to protect French hearts from foie gras, butter, and creamy sauces, researchers continue to ponder over what actually accounts for this seeming paradox.

One famous French investigation that erodes the cholesterol theory is the Lyon Diet Heart Study, published in the late 1990s. It showed that heart attack survivors following a Mediterranean diet were far less likely to experience a second heart attack, unstable angina, heart failure, or cardiac-related death than individuals on the typical low-fat diet endorsed by the American Heart Association. At the study's conclusion, the French researchers found similar cholesterol levels in both groups, but something in the Mediterranean diet clearly protected participants from heart disease. Perhaps it was the important antioxidants in fruits and vegetables or the generous amounts of the anti-inflammatory omega-3 fatty acids from fish and fish oil.

Those relevant studies point to the fact that high cholesterol is not the killer it has been made out to be. The tragedy, though, is that the United States and the rest of the Western world has become obsessed with removing a substance from the body that nature intended us to have. Because of this obsession, many medical professionals worry only about cholesterol and ignore the other risk factors for CVD.

In New Cardiology, we regard cholesterol as detrimental only when it becomes oxidized and contributes to the inflammatory cascade. For sure, it plays a role, but there are a lot of things you can do to keep oxidation in check. More important than reducing cholesterol is defusing other risk factors that ignite and feed the inflammation–plaque process.

Chapter 3

The "Dirty Dozen" Risk Factors

1. Too Much Insulin

Newly diagnosed patients with type 2 diabetes have often had the disease for a decade. By then, many have already sustained long-term endothelial and blood vessel damage, a common characteristic of both diabetes and a prediabetic condition known as insulin resistance.

Some 20 to 25 million Americans are insulin resistant. This sneaky condition does not generate overt symptoms. However, the cells of the body no longer respond normally to insulin, the hormone produced by the pancreas that brings blood sugar (glucose) and fat (triglycerides) into the cells to be used for energy. When this process starts failing, the pancreas compensates by releasing more insulin, but it doesn't work well. The end result is high blood sugar and diabetes. Ample insulin exists in the system, but cell membranes no longer respond to the insulin signal. Glucose and triglycerides cannot enter the cells. Consequently, they build up in the circulation.

Over time, the high tide of blood sugar and insulin wreak havoc on the body and blood vessels by orchestrating a chain reaction of biochemical developments that sets the stage for silent arterial inflammation. Those events include:

- Raised CRP level.
- Thicker and stickier blood—an unheralded risk factor for CVD.

- Increased clotting tendency in the blood.
- Proliferation of smooth muscle tissue in blood vessel walls, contributing to the formation of plaque.
- Free radical damage to cells.
- Protein glycation, in which glucose abnormally binds to healthy proteins in the bloodstream or in the matrix of arterial walls.
- Blood vessel spasm and constriction.
- Increased vascular resistance, contributing to high blood pressure. The higher your blood sugar, the higher your blood pressure and the faster you age.
- Carbohydrates being stored as fat. Translation: weight gain.

All those effects add up to a lot of damage, which is why we regard insulin resistance and its blood test marker—elevated insulin—as powerful indicators of inflammation and CVD.

One obvious sign of an insulin problem is being overweight and shaped a bit like an apple. That means you are packing too much interior abdominal fat, which acts like a gland, releasing a number of proinflammatory substances. For men, waists should be less than 40 inches; for women, less than 35 inches.

2. Toxic Blood

In New Cardiology, toxic blood describes sick blood filled with elements that either contribute to or indicate the presence of arterial inflammation and plaque formation. All these substances can be measured by your doctor.

Homocysteine

Homocysteine, an amino acid, triggers arterial plaque and blood clot formation when it exceeds normal physiologic levels in the body. Kilmer McCully, chief of pathology and laboratory medicine service in the Boston Veterans Administration Health Care System, is the father of the homocysteine theory, a revolutionary explanation of how arterial disease develops.

"In the production of plaques in the artery wall, it is well known that cholesterol becomes damaged by oxidation," McCully says. "But homocysteine is a potent catalyst for this oxidation reaction and orchestrates all the things in the arterial wall that produce the plaque. It orchestrates the thrombosis, the oxidation of the cholesterol lipids and proteins, and participates in virtually all the pathogenic processes that produce atherosclerotic plaques."

Protein is a basic part of all food. One of its primary constituents is methionine, an essential dietary amino acid needed for proper growth and maintenance of all the cells and tissues in the body. Normally, the liver processes methionine and breaks it down into homocysteine, another amino acid. The body recycles some of this homocysteine back into methionine again for protein use throughout the system. Unused homocysteine is excreted in the urine.

This thrifty operation depends on three B-complex vitamins: folic acid, B-6, and B-12. They are necessary cofactors for the enzymes that detoxify. Enzymes are specialized proteins that perform biochemical reactions.

Without enough B-complex vitamins in the diet, homocysteine starts building up in the body and becomes drawn into the endothelial cells. It is believed that the pathogenic sequence of chemical and oxidative reactions is then initiated, encouraging the formation of blood clots.

Studies show that homocysteine is a prime causative agent in 20 to 40 percent of patients with arterial disease. It is especially treacherous in the company of high Lp(a), which we will discuss next. They both promote plaque initiation, progression, and rupture.

Lipoprotein(a)

As we have discussed, Lp(a) performs basic repair duties in the arterial walls. However, when inflammation develops, it can overwhelm the natural healing mechanisms and clog up arteries.

Genetics influences the amount of Lp(a) in your blood. If Lp(a) has been a problem for your family, ask your doctor to test you.

In the presence of a vitamin C deficiency, Lp(a) can become an exceptionally dangerous risk factor. The late Linus Pauling, a two-time Nobel Prize winner, believed that Lp(a) arterial repair becomes relegated to a secondary role when the body contains a plentiful amount of vitamin C. That's because the vitamin serves as an essential raw material for the manufacture of strong collagen—the structural protein that makes up connective tissue, including arterial tissue. With little vitamin C in the system, collagen's ability to maintain and repair tissue suffers. The tissue that comprises blood vessels, both large and small, becomes weak and more easily damaged.

Pauling felt that Lp(a) evolved to serve as a temporary patch during periods of vitamin C deficiency. Today, because of poor diet and the free radical overload associated with modern life, vitamin C deficiency is not uncommon. In a deficiency state, Lp(a) is constantly being pulled in to the artery wall, contributing to progressive atherosclerosis. Pauling contended that the combination of high Lp(a) and vitamin C deficiency creates the most potent underlying cause of atherosclerosis.

A high Lp(a) level—above 30 mg/dl, as determined by a blood test— is reason for great concern. That's because milligram for milligram, Lp(a) has ten times the plaque-producing potential of oxidized LDL.

Lp(a) increases in unstable diabetics and some menopausal women. This may be one reason why the incidence of heart disease quadruples among older women. Conversely, Lp(a) decreases with estrogen replacement therapy.

No prescriptions adequately counteract Lp(a). Nor do dietary cholesterol reduction and exercise. Moreover, cholesterol-lowering statin drugs compound the problem. They may *increase* Lp(a).

Unfortunately, most cardiologists do not test for Lp(a). Most patients who see us for recurrent or inoperable angina have an elevated (and previously unrecognized) Lp(a) level. This explains why their bypass grafts close down and why their arteries renarrow following angioplasty. Studies show a connection between high Lp(a) and poor outcomes following bypass surgery or angioplasty, and continued problems among individuals with unstable angina and a background of heart attack.

C-Reactive Protein

Recent research has identified C-reactive protein (CRP), an antibody-like blood protein, as a formidable indicator and mediator of heart attack and stroke risk. The CRP level rises with chronic infection, high blood sugar, overweight status, and antioxidant and essential fatty acid deficiency. Any one of these situations produces proinflammatory substances such as CRP, ratcheting up the chances for developing atherosclerosis.

CRP may rise transiently with any infection, such as when you battle the flu or a urinary tract infection. The level falls after recovery. We worry about a persistent elevation in CRP, reflecting a continuing and inappropriate inflammation such as arterial inflammation.

Various aspects of insulin resistance are associated with increased CRP, particularly waist circumference. Inner abdominal fat generates interleukin-6, a protein that stimulates the liver to produce CRP.

Fibrinogen

Fibrinogen is a coagulation-regulating protein that converts into fibrin, the fibrous substance that binds with aggregated platelets to form clots. It also determines the stickiness and viscosity of your blood. At a normal level, it promotes the clotting necessary to stop bleeding when you've been injured. But too much of this otherwise good thing is dangerous. It makes blood clot faster—too fast, in fact, which can cause a cardiovascular event.

A higher-than-normal level of fibrinogen represents an independent risk factor for CVD, stroke, sudden death, and restenosis following angioplasty or stent implantation. The tendency toward a high level may be genetic.

Smoking raises fibrinogen significantly. If you smoke, get tested. Elevated fibrinogen—over 350 mg/dl—is a clear warning to stop smoking unless you are looking for trouble. Insulin resistance also contributes to higher fibrinogen.

In women younger than forty-five, we see more heart attacks caused by improper blood clotting. Younger females taking the birth-control pill should also be tested, as well as older women, because fibrinogen rises as estrogen declines.

Ferritin

The body requires iron to make hemoglobin, the red blood cell pigment that carries oxygen to the cells. But recent research suggests that iron excess—more than you need to make hemoglobin—contributes to CVD in different ways. Too much can oxidize LDL cholesterol, rendering it more likely to layer out as plaque. Too much also poisons the endothelial cells and promotes inflammation.

In the early 1980s, Jerome Sullivan, a clinical assistant professor of pathology at the University of Florida, noticed that women who had undergone hysterectomies had increased incidence of heart disease. He suggested that if losing blood protected menstruating women, men donating blood might also have similar protection. His findings clashed head-on with the cholesterol-is-the-cause paradigm and only recently have his theories been accepted.

Menstruating women produce estrogen, which is heart protective, and most lose a significant amount of iron in the blood each month. In contrast, postmenopausal women are four times more likely to have heart attacks. They lose their estrogen protection and also the protection of regular iron release through menstruation. The level of ferritin begins to soar after menopause.

For men, this is an issue as well. In 1992, a five-year Finnish study of nineteen hundred men, aged forty-two to sixty, reported that those with ferritin levels above 200 µg/L were more than twice as likely to have a heart attack. And if their LDL cholesterol was also elevated (the cutoff in this study was LDL above 193 mg/dl), the risk increased five-fold. This makes sense. Elevated ferritin reflects excess iron, an oxidizing factor. LDL cholesterol is the stuff that oxidizes to produce plaque. The combination is deadly.

If you experience fatigue and complain to your doctor, he or she might prescribe iron, the last thing you need if you are already in iron overload. Before you take an iron supplement, insist that your physician give you a serum ferritin test.

3. Oxidative Stress

Free radicals are atoms with one electron as opposed to the normal two electrons in their outer shell. Unstable and reactive, free radicals seek another electron to become stable. A free radical snatches an electron from an adjacent atom, quenching its own electron thirst but damaging the neighboring atom, thus creating a new free radical. A chain reaction can occur, and when enough atoms become damaged, the molecule containing them becomes damaged. Free radicals attack DNA, leading to dysfunction, mutation, and cancer. They attack enzymes and proteins, causing malfunction of normal cell activities. If enough molecules become damaged, the section of the cell containing them becomes damaged. If free radicals damage mitochondria, the structures inside cells where energy production takes place, cells lose vitality. If they attack an LDL cholesterol particle, the particle can become oxidized.

Unchecked free radical stress accelerates aging and age-related degenerative diseases. The domino effect of free radicals, first theorized more than thirty years ago by Denham Harman, a University of Nebraska researcher, is the most widely accepted scientific explanation for aging. His free radical theory of aging holds that free radicals are causal factors in nearly every known disease as well as in the aging process itself. Harman has repeatedly said that aging changes are induced by free radical reactions largely initiated by the mitochondria and that the rate of damage to the mitochondria determines life span.

Chain reactions instigated by electron-hungry atoms go on everywhere all the time. A veritable center court of free radical activity is none other than the vital microscopic organs inside cells called mitochondria, where cellular energy is produced. Our cells utilize oxygen atoms to make energy. One by-product of this ongoing process is the constant creation of a huge number of free radicals. Researchers say this nonstop bioenergetic process can itself generate a trillion oxygen free radicals in each cell. This poses a serious threat to the mitochondria and to cell survival.

Every puff on a cigarette brings a load of free radicals and cadmium (a toxic metal) into the bloodstream to damage the endothelium. Lighting up can temporarily narrow arteries an additional 5 percent. Not that we condone smoking, but if you take vitamin C beforehand, you'll get some protection from cigarette spasm.

Free radicals are also generated by high sugar intake, excessive physical or emotional stress, heavy metal toxins, medical radiation, trans fats, certain drugs, and the immune system's response to chronic infection. The oxidative stress inflicted by free radicals on tissues is similar to the oxidation of metal (rusting) or the oxidation of a fat such as butter (turning it rancid).

Antioxidant compounds made by your cells eliminate free radicals. You also get antioxidants from food, notably fruits and vegetables, and supplements. It's when free radicals are not contained at a tolerable level by antioxidants that they set off their destructive blitz of oxidation.

4. Poor Bioenergetics

Mitochondria generate energy in a complex process called bioenergetics that involves enzymes, protons, electrons, and electrical charges. For the sake of simplicity, we can say a cell membrane opens its doors to gather in oxygen, along with sugars and fatty acids derived from food, and dispatches them to the mitochondria. There, the raw materials are processed by enzymes to make a substance called adenosine triphosphate, or ATP. ATP acts like a high-octane fuel to power all the cells in the body.

Cells contain between two hundred and five thousand mitochondria each. When they don't function properly, an energy crisis develops, spreading disorder and inefficiency throughout the body. Brain, heart, and muscle cells, the heaviest consumers of energy, fail to carry out their basic functions as nature intended. Tissues begin to degenerate.

Heart muscle cells are packed with mitochondria. In fact, they make up about a third of the volume of these cells, more than any tissue in the body. That's obviously nature's way of generating the power necessary to stoke the heart's round-the-clock pumping action over a lifetime.

The heart becomes extremely vulnerable as a result of reduced oxygen and energy due to arterial inflammation and occlusive plaque. Anything that can restore cellular energy in patients with angina, heart failure, left ventricular enlargement, or even hypertension is a great boon. Three very important nutritional supplements are effective: CoQ10, L-carnitine, and D-ribose. They directly support ATP production and thus defend heart cells from the ravages of aging, toxins, and the many conditions that wear down mitochondrial function and cause CVD.

5. The Bacterial Threat

Gum Disease

For many people, heart disease may begin in the mouth. We frequently see this connection in patients with missing and loose teeth, pus pockets, and even foul breath. We can tell a lot about patients just by looking in their mouths.

Gum disease is not a minor problem, or even one localized to the mouth. Numerous studies show a definite connection to heart disease risk, and those with the most serious infections are the ones at greatest risk.

In 1998, the American Academy of Periodontology issued a strong warning that gum infections represent a "far more serious threat" to the health of millions of Americans than previously realized. They cited an increased risk for heart disease, stroke, and underweight births.

Gum disease is an infectious, inflammatory condition caused by bacteria. The infections, which can last for decades, place enormous stress on the immune system. Inflammatory compounds and poisonous waste materials from destroyed bacteria (endotoxins) circulate throughout the body, creating a hyperimmune and systemic inflammatory state.

Typically, bacteria entering the bloodstream are killed and eliminated. But people with serious infections, existing heart disease, or compromised immune systems due to diabetes and respiratory diseases have a lesser ability to fight bacteria.

In the bloodstream, periodontal bacteria can invade susceptible

The Bad Gums Epidemic

- Nine out of ten adults have gingivitis (inflamed gums), which leads to tooth loss if not controlled.
- More than two-thirds of teenagers and a third of younger children already have mild gingivitis.
- Two out of ten adults suffer from destructive periodontitis—advanced gum disease.
- One out of ten adults has no natural teeth. Many more are missing multiple teeth.

arteries. The bloodstream swarms with antibodies against these common oral microorganisms. But as the disease progresses, the antibodies also attack damaged arterial tissue.

In one fascinating study, researchers monitored the starting oral health of ten thousand then-healthy individuals aged twenty-five to seventy-four and correlated it to their cardiovascular health over the next fourteen years. Subjects with a pristine mouth had a 10 percent risk of CVD. If they had gingivitis at baseline, the risk was 14 percent. Periodontitis sent the risk soaring to 32 percent. If all the teeth were out, 42 percent!

Nanobacteria

Nanobacterium sanguineum. Nanobacteria for short. They are only a hundredth the size of normal bacteria and have the distinction of being the smallest cell-walled organisms known on the planet. Until recently, only a few scientists believed anything that small could actually be alive. They are very much alive, and dangerous, and present in all of us, floating through the bloodstream, then infiltrating tissue.

To protect themselves from our immune defenses, nanobacteria envelop themselves in a slimy, impenetrable calcific biofilm, where they very slowly multiply and expand. This slow reproduction means that they may be in the body for many years before they can have an appreciable effect on inflammation and plaque formation. They burrow into healthy cells and cause them to die. The toxicity of the biofilm stimulates an unsuccessful but persistent immune reaction that generates inflammatory chemicals such as CRP. Nanobacteria calcify the environment they live in, and thus contribute over time to the destruction of arterial walls, arthritic joints, and kidney tissue.

Two Finnish researchers, Olavi Kajander and Neva Ciftcioglu, of the University of Kuopio, discovered nanobacteria in 1988. Subsequently, they have theorized that calcific plaques plugging our arteries result from longstanding infection.

More research is needed to validate this idea. But it reminds us of the discovery by J. Robin Warren and Barry Marshall, two medical researchers in Australia, that peptic ulcer disease was due to a bacterial infection. Before this breakthrough, doctors were convinced that ulcers were due to too much stomach acid. Now we treat ulcers with antibiotics. The Australians' discovery won the Nobel Prize in 2005.

One frightening hypothesis is that nanobacteria enter the body via common vaccines manufactured with fetal bovine serum, a breeding ground for these bacteria. Recent studies have shown that early plaque deposition can be detected in males twenty years and younger. We blame the epidemic of early-onset coronary disease on diet, stress, and smoking. Could the increasing number of vaccines being administered to youngsters also lead to premature atherosclerosis?

Many nanobacteria questions exist for which we have no answers yet, but we appear to have a new theory for the calcification process accompanying prolonged inflammation, plaque formation, and the aging process. European studies have found these microorganisms present in more than 60 percent of artery-clogging plaques in different parts of the body.

6. Toxic Metals

When Emperor Nero fiddled while Rome burned in A.D. 64, it probably wasn't that he didn't care for the plight of the Roman capital but rather that he couldn't care because his brain had been addled by lead. Lead is a biological poison. Then, and now, it has no place in the body.

The Romans made extensive use of it in daily life, in cosmetics, plumbing, and painting. Roman wine was contaminated with lead due to the practice of simmering grape syrup in lead vessels to enhance flavor. Historians speculate that infertility and mental infirmity due to lead poisoning from excessive wine consumption figured in the decline of Roman civilization. Perhaps an explanation for Nero's behavior.

Today, we extract a billion tons of lead a year from the earth's crust,

Mercury enters the body via contaminated air, fish, dental fillings, and vaccines. We believe that you cannot neutralize mercury without adequate selenium. This is one reason why supplementation is so important.

7. Emotional Stress

When you are fired up emotionally, you're putting a torch to your arteries. Medical research has repeatedly documented the danger of anger, chronic stress, and the negative emotional states associated with depression and social isolation. We have clearly seen the heavy toll that psychological status and emotions take on patients. These are hidden risk factors rarely addressed by doctors. For instance:

- Chronic anger contributes to high blood pressure and heart enlargement. Acute situational anger can promote clot formation.
- Depression significantly increases the risk of heart disease. Among other effects, it actually triples the disease-producing effect of smoking.
- Lack of a social support network fuels atherosclerosis. Little or no support after a heart attack translates into a three- to four-time greater risk of premature death than if patients are surrounded by friends and family.

Modern medicine has explained many of the physiological relationships of the mind/body connection. In the early 1900s, Harvard physiologist Walter Cannon first described the fight-or-flight response—the internal response of the body to a threat or a perceived threat. The body releases stress hormones that touch off a cascade of events priming a person or an animal to run or fight. This mechanism served well for cavemen facing saber-toothed tigers, but most of the threats we face in modern life tend to be psychological and cannot be handled by fighting or fleeing. At Canada's McGill University in the 1950s, Hans Selye, the world's foremost authority on stress, demonstrated that the body reacts to modern-day stressors as though it were still facing the same physical threat as our early ancestors.

Under chronic stress—for example, constant deadlines, a rocky marriage, an unfulfilling job—your body secretes excess cortisol, a stress hormone. Growing evidence indicates that overproduction of this and related hormones plays a major role in a wide variety of illnesses, including CVD. The hormones promote arterial constriction, high blood pressure, and increased heart rate.

Stress also causes the blood to clot more. This serves the soldier exposed to life-and-death combat situations. You want more clotting should you become wounded. The clotting slows down or plugs up blood loss.

However, the equivalent of daily combat in the office or a fractious relationship generates a similar process in the body. The blood becomes more the consistency of red ketchup than red wine, an analogy created by cardiologist Kenneth R. Kensey, a pioneer in the study of blood viscosity (thickness and stickiness) as a risk factor for CVD. The thicker and stickier the blood becomes, the greater the risk for cardiovascular problems.

Stress reactions are largely governed by the *autonomic nervous system* (ANS), a branch of the nervous system over which we usually have no direct voluntary control. It, in turn, has two components: the *sympathetic nervous system* (SNS), which causes the arousal responses previously described, and the *parasympathetic nervous system* (PNS), which calms and relaxes the body. Most stress management techniques, including meditation and biofeedback, aim to induce a positive parasympathetic state by calming down an SNS constantly in overdrive.

In the 1960s, cardiologists Meyer Friedman and Ray Rosenman, of the Mount Zion Medical Center in San Francisco, identified a cluster of overdrive behavior—constant hurriedness, hostility, and intense competitiveness—that seemed to characterize many of their patients with heart disease. They coined the term *type A behavior* to describe those individuals, and the name soon became common.

Over the years, researchers have recognized that hurriedness and competitiveness are less damaging to the heart than hostility. People prone to hostility show much longer increases in blood pressure and stress hormones.

Did you know that accountants die from heart attacks more during tax season because their oxidized cholesterol goes way up due to stress? And did you know that the single largest incidence of heart attacks—28 percent—occur on Monday morning? Cardiologists call this phenomenon Monday morning syndrome. Recently, researchers at Tokyo Women's Medical University also found that many workers suffer a spike in blood pressure as they return to the office after the weekend.

Occupational statistics reveal job dissatisfaction among more than three-quarters of people in the workforce. If going to work on Monday is like going into battle, then no wonder that heart attacks occur en masse at this time.

By the way, Saturday runs second in this dubious category—14 percent of heart attacks occur on that day. A combat zone at home could certainly account for the Saturday spike.

An Israeli researcher reported in 2004 on a study of two hundred patients who had experienced a mini-stroke (transient ischemic attack, or TIA). The investigation showed that anger and intense negative emotions could increase the risk of stroke by as much as fourteen times.

In 2002, cardiologists at the University Hospital in Zurich found that mental stress causes the inner layer of the blood vessels to constrict, which may increase the risk of a heart attack or a stroke. Their study provided the first evidence that mental stress induces endothelial dysfunction.

Stress takes many forms. Doctors frequently see heartbreak and grief—such as the loss of a spouse or a stressful career—translate into heart disease. Heartache can eventually lead to heartbreak, or the literal breaking down of heart function.

8. Gender Factors

Hormones are messenger molecules that govern physiology—the way your body functions. Secreted by glands such as the adrenals, testes, ovaries, and thyroid, these specialized proteins flash through your blood-stream carrying instructions to the cells. Cell membranes are outfitted with multiple gates called receptor sites. Hormones reach specific target cells, unlock their respective gates, and deliver their biochemical message to DNA (deoxyribonucleic acid) for processing. So they regulate specific cellular functions, as well as monitor cellular activity throughout the system.

Glands produce larger or smaller amounts of different hormones at different times of the day, month, and stage of life, and according to your activities. The levels of nearly all those hormones start to decline after you reach your midtwenties.

Estrogen in women and testosterone in men are sex hormones that provide specific cardiovascular protection. Low estrogen and low testosterone that accompany aging are associated with inflammatory states. Low testosterone makes men more likely to clot and develop atherosclerosis. The same goes for estrogen in women after menopause. These are independent risk factors.

Moreover, we know that certain chemicalized hormones, such as progestins like Provera (a synthetic progesterone drug replacement for women), can be harmful to the heart. Progestins were introduced years ago to prevent the overgrowth of endometrial tissue and to lower the risk of uterine cancer that could occur from estrogen monotherapy.

Today, growing numbers of cardiologists are openly warning doctors about Provera. Specifically, the drug is coronary constrictive, which means it reduces the diameter of the arteries leading to the heart.

Unfortunately, women who take the synthetic hormone replacements routinely prescribed for years put themselves at higher risk for heart attack and stroke. This was clearly demonstrated in the large Women's Health Initiative Study halted in midstream with much media attention in 2003, because the risk had become so obvious. Today, cardiologists oppose routine hormone replacement therapy because of the documented danger to the cardiovascular system. Recent studies suggest that short-term hormone replacement early in menopause may have some cardiovascular benefits, but the cardiology jury is still undecided.

9. Trans-Fatty Acids

Naturally occurring oils in food are good fats that your body needs. And there are bad fats that you definitely don't need.

The biggest troublemakers are man-made partially hydrogenated fats. They start life as polyunsaturated vegetable oils, usually corn and canola. Food processors bubble hydrogen through them and turn them into solid fats such as margarine and shortening. The objective: a stable fat with a long shelf life—great for manufacturers but not for us.

Remember the cookies your grandmother made? They were stale after three days. Today's cookies live practically forever, soft and chewy, because of partially hydrogenated oils. An estimated 75 percent of foods eaten in the standard American diet contain these fats: most packaged baked goods, fried snacks, frozen products such as fish sticks and french fries, some brands of peanut butter, microwave popcorn, commercial salad dressings, and pancake mixes. The list goes on and on.

The hydrogenation process creates trans-fatty acids—trans fats for short—unnatural chemicals associated with increased free radical damage to cell membranes. Cellular damage of this sort kindles inflammation, disease, and age-related changes. These fats raise Lp(a), promote LDL oxidation, and lower HDL. In short, they ignite CVD.

Nutrition experts at Harvard make the connection quite clear: "By our most conservative estimate, replacement of partially hydrogenated fat in the U.S. diet with natural unhydrogenated vegetable oils would prevent approximately 30,000 premature coronary deaths per year, and epidemiologic evidence suggests this number is closer to 100,000."

These fats also show up in many fried foods, because the high heat involved in frying leads to the partial decomposition of fat and the formation of toxic by-products. The high heat can even damage stable saturated fats such as lard and butter.

Trans fats harm enzymes including delta-6-desaturase, which converts beneficial dietary fats (see discussion of dietary fats in chapter 9) to forms used by the body. In this way, trans fats can actually escalate essential fatty acid deficits. This is an important but overlooked issue. We ingest fish oils and convert them into health-nurturing substances. But not if we eat trans fats! The same enzymes that convert good fats recognize trans fats as if they were wholesome, allowing them into their receptor sites where they stick and destroy the enzymes. The enzymes are then unable to manufacture healthy prostaglandins, fatty acids with hormone-like properties that help regulate pain, fever, inflammation, vascular tone, clotting, and blood pressure. Instead, trans fats turn on ugly prostaglandins, and these inflammatory agents poison the vascular system. Overloading on trans fats nullifies the good fats you eat or take as supplements. Trans fats prevent you from using the good oils to protect your health. They are metabolic poison.

Dietary guidelines tell us that no more than 1 percent of our caloric intake should come from trans fats. A small order of fast-food restaurant french fries contains a day-and-a-half's worth of trans fats. A 2002 report from a National Academy of Sciences panel concluded that "the only safe intake of trans-fat is zero."

We applaud the U.S. Food and Drug Administration for making manufacturers disclose trans fat content on the labels of food products starting in 2006. We also applaud those fast-food restaurant chains that have eliminated trans fats. We hope that trans fats might someday be banned altogether. For more information on trans fats, see the special report on the Web site of the Center for Science in the Public Interest (www.cspinet.org).

10. High Blood Pressure

Hypertension, or high blood pressure as it is commonly known, is not really a disease. It is a by-product of other, often more serious, underlying problems, resulting in excessive force of blood pressing against the walls of the arteries. Fully one-third of individuals with high blood pressure have no symptoms and don't even know they have it.

High blood pressure leads to cardiovascular disaster: heart attack, heart failure, stroke, brain damage, and kidney disease. Uncontrolled hypertension, in fact, ranks as the leading risk factor for heart attack and stroke, with women even more vulnerable to its ravages than men.

In 90 percent of cases, known as essential hypertension, the cause remains unknown. Among the causal factors are age, body weight, diet, heredity, ethnicity (high blood pressure affects more blacks than whites), kidney infection, and stress.

High blood pressure conspires with all the other risk factors—cigarette smoke, oxidized LDL, Lp(a), and toxic metals. The condition literally pounds these toxins into the artery walls, weakens blood vessels at the bends and splits, and accelerates the inflammatory–plaque cascade.

Moreover, hypertension stimulates the release of two proteins, angiotensin II and endothelin, which further promote and accelerate inflammatory and oxidative mechanisms in arteries. The evidence suggests that this inflammation may be the direct connection between hypertension and atherosclerosis.

High Blood Pressure by the Numbers

A person is considered to have high blood pressure if he or she has a systolic pressure of 140 mmHg or greater and/or a diastolic pressure of 90 mmHg or greater, or is taking antihypertensive medication. Systolic means the pressure when the heart contracts. Diastolic means the pressure between heartbeats when the heart relaxes. A normal blood pressure is 120 over 80 or less.

---

11. Genetics

Recent decades have brought exciting advances and understanding about the role of genetics in illness. For cardiologists, the Human Genome Project, which has mapped the location and role of various genes, has opened new doors to the diagnosis and treatment of CVD. When people say "it's a family thing" referring to somebody's illness, we are now starting to have specifics about what that means. And along with the specifics come better solutions.

Take the case of Sid as an example. He had successful coronary artery bypass surgery in the late 1990s and had been enjoying a good quality of life ever since. But he continued to have high blood pressure. His family had a history of it, and with this stubborn problem, his risk for another cardiac event was great, even though he felt fine.

Dr. Sinatra individualized a protocol of supplements, medication, and lifestyle changes for Sid. But his hypertension didn't drop. A genetic profile blood test provided a clue—the presence of two alleles (specific combinations of genes) indicating that androgens (male hormones) and estrogens might be responsible for Sid's high blood pressure. In this case, the testosterone he was taking for his decreased libido appeared to be the culprit.

The results suggested that testosterone could interfere with his medication and even keep pushing the blood pressure up. Even though Sid was pleased with the libido benefits of the hormone, he agreed to stop the testosterone for the sake of his overall health. Before long, his blood pressure numbers began to steadily go down.

Clearly, the genetic profile helped solve the mystery. Insurance companies don't pay for this state-of-the-art test (it costs about $300), so it is not something we order routinely. Nevertheless, we both feel that genetic testing should not be overlooked, particularly in tough, resistant cases.

12. Radiation

We are all exposed to radiation in the form of medical X-rays. Cardiologists, for instance, are exposed to a considerable amount of radiation because of the nature of this work. We do fluoroscopy all the time, putting in pacemakers and cardiac catheterizations. Fluoroscopy uses X-rays to view parts of the body on a screen, similar to the screening your luggage undergoes when you pass through airport security.

No strong evidence exists that radiation damages the heart, yet we suspect there is a cardiovascular connection. Radiation can damage DNA in the X-ray path and literally cause plaque because such damage can set off inflammation. When you are being radiated, you are essentially being burned.

About five years ago, Dr. Sinatra was perplexed to find out that despite all his personal preventive health practices, he had highly oxidized LDL. After searching for possible causes, he came to the conclusion that work-related radiation had done the damage.

We both have had patients with non-Hodgkin's lymphoma who received radiation in the chest and then developed coronary disease. In cardiology, we call that radiation atherosclerosis. We believe X-rays damage endothelial cells. A prime example was a patient with multiple risk factors for CVD, including diabetes and high blood pressure. In 1995, prior to beginning New Cardiology therapy, he was treated with radiation for a neck tumor. Subsequent diagnosis revealed 35 percent narrowings in both his carotid arteries. Eight years later, carotid ultrasound showed substantial deterioration with high-grade obstruction. Yet a coronary angiogram revealed clean arteries in the heart, an area not exposed to the radiation beam. The conclusion was that the head and neck radiation had damaged the carotid endothelium, promoting plaque formation, while the treatment program prevented plaque buildup in the coronaries. We normally expect arterial disease in the carotids to be accompanied by some coronary disease.

We have patients asking for unnecessary chest X-rays every year. Don't get more X-rays than you need. If your doctor says X-rays are necessary, that's another thing. But X-rays do have a downside. Too many raise the risk of endothelial or DNA damage, chronic inflammation, and cancer, whether it's mammograms, dental X-rays, CT scans, or cardiology angiograms. Multiple angiograms on a patient may promote disease progression. No research shows this, but we tread very conservatively on this issue.

Radiation abounds in our present-day environment. Radiation damage accumulates and doesn't disappear from your body. If you have been exposed to excessive radiation in your neck and heart area, be very prudent about reducing your overall CVD risk factors.

In 2006, a report from radiation oncology researchers at the University of Pennsylvania caught our attention. Their research involved a laboratory experiment showing that antioxidants effectively protected human breast epithelial cells against a variety of radiation-induced free radical damage. The specific cell line they used is a standard research model used in cancer studies.

The cells were treated before and after radiation exposure with a combination of the following antioxidants: N-acetylcysteine, vitamin C (ascorbic acid and sodium ascorbate), CoQ10, alpha-lipoic acid, selenium (1-selenomethionine), and vitamin E. These substances are all commonly available as nutritional supplements in health food stores. The researchers concluded that antioxidants appear to be "promising" countermeasures for protection from adverse biologic effects caused by radiation.

PART TWO

How to Get Unclogged

Chapter 4

Tests You Need

A middle-aged dentist with a family history of cardiovascular disease and sudden death made an appointment after one of our lectures. He wanted a full screen of his blood—all the New Cardiology risk factors. The results revealed a high degree of coronary artery calcium buildup, high Lp(a), homocysteine, and fibrinogen.

The dentist was distraught when he heard the news. "How do we get rid of this plaque? I'll do anything," he said.

Unfortunately, we can't scrape it off like we would do with dental plaque. In order to get rid of it or defuse it, we first have to find out what causes it.

Even though arterial disease is 90 percent silent—you don't have any symptoms—and half the time sudden death is the first symptom, our broadened New Cardiology approach has dramatically ramped up our ability to decipher and overcome the enemy.

For years, physicians have been doing routine blood tests assessing total cholesterol, HDL, LDL, triglycerides, and blood sugar. For the most part, doctors are still fixated on cholesterol numbers and the simplistic concept of LDL as the "bad" cholesterol and HDL as the "good" stuff. But this standard screening doesn't cut it anymore.

Patients whose arteries continue to clog despite appropriate lipid (LDL, HDL, and triglyceride) control often come to us for a second opinion. We are continually appalled to discover that those measurements are the only CVD risk factors they have had tested. Even more disturbing are the heavy-duty medications these patients take based on such insufficient data—medications creating overtly dangerous or subtle and insidious side effects.

It's a big lie and a shameful disservice to the public when the pharmaceutical industry and doctors project a happy face of cardiac protection if you swallow a cholesterol-lowering drug every day. That's hardly the best that can be offered to prevent heart disease.

Silent inflammation is the root cause of CVD. Although there are many sophisticated blood tests to detect toxic blood substances, those tests are often not covered by health insurance. For example, Lp(a) is one of the most virulent cardiovascular risk factors, but some insurance companies refuse to cover the cost of this test.

This is especially infuriating because today's technology provides cardiologists with tests to make highly accurate predictions and follow up with specifically targeted treatment. Unlike cancer, still in the primitive stage when it comes to making predictions and arresting a budding cancerous process before it becomes a life-threatening tumor, our specialty has many tests—exciting new ones and dependable old ones—to uncover risks.

For years, we have used electrocardiograms (EKGs) and treadmill stress tests. And with those we could determine in a general way if you had some risk. But we couldn't look you in the eye and say to what degree you were at risk and what elements in the disease process concerned us the most. If your results turned up enough red flags, we performed an invasive angiogram to get a clearer picture of blockage in the coronary arteries. But cardiologists generally hesitate to perform this procedure because it carries risk. Typically, we reserve it for patients with pronounced symptoms or if the noninvasive data indicate a significant probability of obstructive artery disease.

In New Cardiology, we utilize a variety of tests to pinpoint problems before resorting to an invasive procedure. The diagnosis of cardiovascular-related illnesses has produced astounding advances in recent years, allowing us to detect and treat the early signs of potentially lethal cardiovascular situations before they become serious. We have the tools today to avert the danger, some truly amazing diagnostics readily available to patients. But often doctors are unaware of them.

In this chapter, you will learn about some of these lifesaving tests that we believe hold the key to successful CVD prevention, therapy, and risk factor assessment. We'll cover the standard tests first, then go into detail on new procedures that sharpen the detective work needed to unmask plaque and identify someone at risk for sudden death. We'll look at new blood tests and imaging procedures.

We prescribe individual tests depending on the patient. Some people see us solely with prevention in mind. Some have mild symptoms, like vague discomfort in the chest and slight shortness of breath. Others have outright signs of disease or a family history of premature heart disease. Both of us are conventionally trained cardiologists. If a patient has clear signs of acute cardiovascular distress, we resort to an angiogram right away. Such patients have pronounced chest discomfort; excess sweating; rapid fatigue with exertion; arm, neck, or jaw pain; and shortness of breath. In acute situations, we don't take chances. We leave the detective work for a later date after patients are out of danger. We can then work to reduce the underlying causes and prevent recurrence.

The Standard Tests

Doctors routinely prescribe these tests according to the individual case and their own personal preferences.

Electrocardiogram (EKG)

A resting EKG assesses the electrical activity of your heart at rest, providing precise information about cardiac rhythm and heart rate and indirect information about coronary blood flow and pump action. The test is routinely performed on the first visit to a cardiologist.

Echocardiogram

The echocardiogram is a noninvasive ultrasound exam that records specific geographical areas of the beating heart, revealing blood flow patterns, and allows us to measure wall thickness of the heart's chambers. Dysfunction of one segment reflects a prior heart attack. We can get a good sense of where valves may be too loose and leaky or too tight and restrictive.

Exercise Stress Test (Exercise EKG)

Typically, the exercise EKG is the first diagnostic test used for determining the presence and/or extent of coronary heart disease. You exercise by walking on a motorized treadmill or riding a stationary bicycle as an electrocardiogram tracks the electrical activity of the heart.

Nuclear Stress Test

The nuclear stress test is the "Rolls Royce" of stress tests. This procedure combines the treadmill with images recorded on a sophisticated computerized camera. It gives us a pictorial view of the heart immediately after exercise. A positive finding indicates blood flow restriction in one or more parts of the heart.

Holter Monitor

A Holter monitor is usually worn for twenty-four hours and every heartbeat is recorded during that time period. This test is ordered to identify cardiac arrhythmias and to monitor how well medication is working in order to control the arrhythmias better.

Coronary Angiogram

The coronary angiogram is considered to be the gold standard in evaluating heart disease. It is also the most invasive diagnostic test. A catheter is inserted into an artery in the groin or the arm and guided up to the heart. A special dye is then injected through the catheter into each of the coronary arteries feeding the heart. The dye provides a contrasting color readily visualized by simple X-ray imaging. The images show the severity and precise location of blockages. This test is usually not recommended unless preliminary tests reveal strong evidence of coronary artery blockage. The angiogram (picture) aids the doctor in selecting subsequent treatment, which may include medications, balloon angioplasty, coronary stenting, or coronary artery bypass surgery.

A new scanning technique called 64-slice coronary CT scanning, a noninvasive equivalent of putting a camera inside the coronary arteries and assessing plaque and calcification status, has become available. Someday it will replace invasive angiography. The method provides previously unobtainable visualization of the coronary arteries with much less radiation and risks. If your cardiologist orders a standard angiogram for you, ask if a 64-slice coronary scan can be done instead.

Carotid Angiogram

Carotid angiograms utilize a similar technique to determine the risk of stroke. A carotid angiogram is indicated when a patient is experiencing symptoms of impaired blood flow to the brain and/or has extensive plaque or a high-grade narrowing based on ultrasound detection.

The New Cardiology Tests

Blood Work

As part of a complete physical, physicians always order a complete blood cell count (CBC), electrolytes (sodium, potassium), a chemical profile, and renal function tests. The usual cardiac evaluation will additionally include a lipid panel (total cholesterol, LDL, HDL, triglycerides, and ratios for these lipids).

We cover all these factors. Going beyond cholesterol, we pay special attention to toxic blood syndrome, dangerous inflammatory elevations of homocysteine, Lp(a), ferritin, fibrinogen, and CRP, and the newest measure of silent inflammation—the AA/EPA test (explained later in this chapter).

We look at hormone levels, particularly estrogen, testosterone, and thyroid. Even a slight hypothyroid status increases the risk of CVD because the body needs thyroid hormone to metabolize cholesterol efficiently.

We check metabolic cardiology status—that is, if the cardiovascular system is well energized. Is the pump getting enough raw materials to do its job? Those materials include vital nutrients such as CoQ10, magnesium, and L-carnitine. If pump performance is subpar, we can get a good idea of what to do in the way of simple supplementation.

We consider as a separate entity the cluster of specific characteristics known as metabolic syndrome—a symptomless set of five markers (four blood measurements along with waist girth) that represents a major risk for CVD. If we need further clarification, and particularly in cases in which outcomes are not readily clear or there are high homocysteine and blood pressure levels that are resistant to treatment, we may resort to genetic tests.

The blood tests we recommend and our ideal healthy zone values are listed for your reference. Refer to chapter 12 for our specific strategies on how to improve your test scores.

These tests are based on blood draws your doctor can order from medical laboratories. Some are covered by insurance and some aren't. Check with your doctor's insurance specialist or with your insurance carrier. Keep in mind that normal ranges may vary from laboratory to laboratory and typically reflect the range of values found in 95 percent of Americans, most of whom will eventually die from CVD or cancer. We want better for you.

New Cardiology Blood Work

Blood Component	Your Level	Healthy Zone
CoQ10	_____	1.0–1.8 µg/ml
CRP	_____	<0.8 mg/L
Ferritin (iron)	_____	Women <80 µg/L
	_____	Men <90 µg/L
Fibrinogen	_____	180–350 mg/dl
Homocysteine	_____	<9 µmol/L
Lp(a)	_____	<30 mg/dl
Total cholesterol	_____	125–200 mg/dl
HDL	_____	Women 40–120 mg/dl
	_____	Men 35–70 mg/dl
LDL	_____	70–130 mg/dl
Oxidized LDL	_____	0–650 units
Triglycerides	_____	50–180 mg/dl
AA/EPA ratio	_____	1.5–3.0

Lead, mercury, and other toxic metals (see chapter 8)

TESTS FOR INSULIN RESISTANCE

Fasting blood sugar	_____	<100 mg/dl
Fasting insulin	_____	<17 microunits/L
Hemoglobin A1C	_____	<6% of total HGB

Cutting-edge laboratories that offer comprehensive testing for New Cardiology inflammatory and oxidative stress factors include: Immunosciences Lab Inc., in Beverly Hills, California; Antibody Assay Reference Laboratory in Santa Ana, California; Metametrix Clinical Laboratory in Norcross, Georgia; and Great Smokies Diagnostics Laboratory in Asheville, North Carolina (see appendix A for contact details).

Testing for Iron Overload

The lab test needed to determine your iron level is called serum ferritin. Ferritin is a protein that stores iron in the body. This test, however, is not part of most doctors' routine screening. You have to ask for it—and you should. The normal range for ferritin in the United States is 10–290 µg/L. Let's say your test level comes in at 250. Most doctors, unaware of the iron-inflammation link, would not take action, but a level above 200 doubles your heart attack risk. We feel that a level around 100 is optimal.

An inherited defect leading to excessive iron absorption is widespread in North America, affecting 1 percent of the population and probably about 5 percent of patients with diabetes or CVD. Such individuals test in the 200 to 400 range. In these cases, a combination of blood donations, and if needed, intramuscular deferroxamine iron-binding therapy, can bring down ferritin levels.

Testing for Key Fatty Acids

The new AA/EPA ratio blood test measures the relationship of the inflammatory-causing omega-6 fatty acid arachidonic acid (AA) to the beneficial omega-3 fatty acid eicosapentaenoic acid (EPA). These substances impact the balance of eicosanoids, hormonelike chemicals produced by cells that influence inflammation. Too many carbohydrates and refined sugars provoke an insulin response. Too much insulin accelerates AA production, which in turn promotes proinflammatory and clot-inducing eicosanoids. At the present time, this test can be performed for you without a doctor's prescription at the following facilities: Your Future Health, Tavares, Florida (877-468-6934), and Nutrasource Diagnostics, Inc., of Guelph, Ontario, Canada (877-557-7722). See the laboratory section of appendix A for additional contact information.

Metabolic Syndrome

Metabolic syndrome involves a specific set of measurements that do not by themselves cause symptoms but represent risk factors for CVD, obesity, diabetes, physical frailty, and premature death. Medical experts believe one out of four adults in the overall population and one out of two over the age of fifty have metabolic syndrome and do not know it. Doctors will likely include most of these factors in their assessment, but they usually do not measure waist girth and do not tend to look at these measurements collectively.

You are at risk if you have any three of the following five characteristics:

1. Waist girth more than 35 inches for a woman and more than 40 inches for a male

2. Fasting blood sugar over 100 mg/dl

3. Triglycerides (blood fats) over 150 mg/dl

4. HDL less than 50 mg/dl for a woman and less than 40 mg/dl for a man

5. Blood pressure over 130/85 or someone requiring a blood pressure medication

In New Cardiology, we look beyond the classic five factors and also consider the fasting insulin and hemoglobin A1C levels. These measurements give us additional proof for the presence of metabolic syndrome and insulin resistance:

1. Insulin level greater than 17 microunits/L

2. Hemoglobin AIC higher than 6 percent of total HGB

Genetics

Among the many benefits emerging from the evolving science of genetics are several tests that screen for potential heart and brain problems. With that information we can advise individual patients what they need to do to keep specific genetic risks in check. It's a powerful strategy both for disease prevention and therapy that's going to become more and more prominent in health care.

For example, the blood protein component called apolipoprotein E (APO E) plays an important role in fat metabolism. The three most common alleles (meaning combinations of genes) responsible for producing APO E are called E2, E3, and E4. These units are associated with cholesterol and lipid disorders.

Not everyone has a given allele. The presence of one may indicate risk for a certain condition. We check for specific alleles to help us make treatment decisions.

This is a dynamic field of research. We present a few examples to show how genetic profiling can be of benefit in disease treatment.

APO E2 Allele
Damage from oxidized dietary fats and cholesterol is lowest in people who have the E2 allele and greatest in those with the E4.

APO E3 Allele
Individuals with this allele respond well to regular exercise. If their total cholesterol is high, they respond better to statin drugs than to vitamin B3 (niacin).

APO E4 Allele
People with the E4 allele tend to have higher blood levels of cholesterol, Lp(a), and triglycerides and lower HDL values. One E4 correlates with susceptibility to heart disease; two with risk of developing premature aging disorders such as arterial disease and Alzheimer's disease, especially if total cholesterol and blood pressure are high. E4 people must watch their diet, limiting high-saturated fats such as butter and lard and trans fats (the hydrogenated oils in processed food). Lowering blood pressure and exercising regularly are important.

We recommend a total inflammatory risk profile for patients with this allele because they must make stringent lifestyle changes that support healing. Having two APO E4 alleles, along with a high mercury concentration and a deficiency in the mineral magnesium, represents a heightened risk factor combination for Alzheimer's disease.

Genetic variations can also impair a basic biological process called methylation—that is, turning one bodily chemical into another by adding or removing methyl groups at the molecular level. Methyl groups are one of the most common structural units of organic compounds, consisting of three hydrogen atoms and a carbon atom linked to the remainder of the molecule.

Methylation can turn treacherous homocysteine back into methionine, an essential amino acid. Some experts believe that as much as 40 percent of the population has a mutation in the gene responsible for producing the enzyme methylenetetrahydrofolate reductase. Should you be among them, your body may not efficiently make the conversion. As your homocysteine level climbs, you become more vulnerable to severe oxidative stress and premature aging. This genetic defect is associated with generalized atherosclerosis, coronary artery disease, stroke, Alzheimer's disease, and cervical cancer. High homocysteine can steal years from your life. Taking vitamin B supplements, as we describe in the next chapter, helps keep homocysteine in check.

Genetic testing is not completely foolproof or widely understood by the public, but it should be considered, especially in challenging cases such as in individuals with high blood pressure, clotting tendencies, and homocysteine levels that just don't respond to regular treatment.

The presence of a particular gene or allele offers clues as to whether a patient may respond to a certain diet, medication, or supplement. If you know your genetic profile, including inherent genetic weaknesses, you can take specific steps to neutralize the impact of these weaknesses.

"The great power of this technology is its potential to deliver a personalized risk message to patients who might not otherwise comply with what we as doctors tell them," says Richard M. Delany, a cardiologist in Milton, Massachusetts, who routinely uses genetic testing in his preventive medicine practice. "We can take a swab from your cheek or blood from your arm and send it to a lab that specifically tests for inherited genes that may predispose you, more than somebody else, to make higher LDL cholesterol if you eat a cheeseburger. So now I can go back to you and say, 'John, I know you like cheeseburgers, but your genes don't like them. They have a bad effect on your cholesterol.' We can apply this information to homocysteine and low HDL cholesterol and all sorts of risk factors that link to many different types of diseases. We can begin to talk in terms of what your specific body requires. Maybe exercise won't actually make a big difference for you. But you may have five mutations in your liver that mean you better cut down on well-done cheeseburgers, increase your intake of cruciferous vegetables, avoid exposure to polyaromatic hydrocarbons present in gasoline fumes, and get out of the business you are in because exposure to certain chemicals could increase the risk of certain cancers or accelerated aging.

"People always tend to listen to us more *after* their heart attacks. Now, with genetic testing, people at high risk may be able to better avoid the heart attack by learning and truly realizing what they individually need more or less of in their specific environment and then putting that information into place by choosing a specific lifestyle to accommodate their genes. This is personalized preventive medicine. People listen and are more inclined to take the information seriously. The goal of DNA testing is to identify specific common mutations that are medically relevant and potentially modifiable."

Imaging

There are two remarkable imaging tests we have come to rely on in recent years. The first, electron beam computerized tomography, measures the calcification in your arteries—that is, the hard plaque. The second, carotid artery intima media thickness, assesses the presence of soft, vulnerable plaque. This is the most dangerous plaque with the greatest potential to rupture.

The combined results of these two tests give us a very accurate picture of the plaque situation systemically and help us determine a comprehensive preventive or therapeutic program.

Electron Beam Computerized Tomography

Electron beam computerized tomography (EBT) offers high-resolution images that measure hardened plaque in the coronary arteries. The technology was first introduced in the early 1990s and is proving to be a reliable, noninvasive way to assess heart attack risk. This is the kind of technology that can save hundreds of thousands of lives.

One of the significant risk factors for CAD is the amount of calcium in the coronary arteries. Cardiologists use the term *coronary calcium*, synonymous with *calcified plaques*. This has nothing to do with the calcium you take, for instance, in supplements to build your bones.

Your heart vessels are not like your teeth and bones, which derive their hardness and strength in large part from calcium. Deposits of calcium don't belong in the arterial walls. Calcification indicates excessive oxidative stress or some unhealthy activity going on within the arterial walls that causes plaque to calcify and harden. When calcium builds up, the vessel walls become more irritated and inflamed. Any patchy, irritated area of a vessel wall attracts red blood cells and fatty molecules, triggering an inflammatory sequence.

Measuring calcified plaque has been demonstrated to be a better predictor of substantial heart attack risk than any of the CVD risk factors identified in major studies, for instance, the Framingham Heart Study. Better, it appears, than high blood pressure, high cholesterol levels, obesity, cigarette smoking, diabetes, and physical inactivity. The greater your calcium score, the greater your plaque burden and the greater your risk for experiencing a coronary event. Even more telling is the rate of change in your calcium score over time. On average, coronary calcium progresses at a rate of 40 percent per year. Individuals with static or slowly progressing scores are at lower risk.

Who should have the test: We strongly recommend EBT as a screening tool for hidden, undiagnosed, or silent coronary artery disease, particularly for people who have a strong family history of the disease or who have multiple risk factors. Let's say we have a patient with very high cholesterol or CRP who is unsure about going on a regimen of statin drugs to lower cholesterol, or a female patient with toxic blood and elevated Lp(a) who is concerned about the side effects of estrogen replacement. A low EBT score suggests we follow a conservative approach. A high score, particularly one that is rising rapidly, calls for more aggressive action.

If you already have symptoms, see a cardiologist as soon as possible. Don't wait for an EBT scan.

Pros: EBT is quick and painless and takes only ten minutes. CAT scan pictures of your heart are taken while you lie on a table. There are no dyes or invasive measures involved.

Cons: Unfortunately, most insurance companies don't cover the $400 to $500 cost of an EBT scan yet. However, it looks like reimbursement is coming soon.

This test produces unreliably high calcium scores on individuals who have had bypass operations or stents. The bypassed native vessel, occluded and full of plaque, is being measured, thus contributing to the higher score. A metal stent will also throw off the accuracy. The highest score we ever encountered was in a male patient who had been bypassed. He had a score of 10,000 (see the results explanation below).

EBT is not perfect. There are false positives and false negatives. The scan may indicate significant calcification; however, obstructive coronary disease may not be present. The scan may uncover a situation worth checking out with further testing.

Similarly, a negative result may not account for the presence of uncalcified, soft coronary plaques in the arteries. These plaques, as we have explained, pose a real danger because they have greater potential to rupture and cause arterial blockage than calcified coronary plaque. We have seen blocked vessels in patients with low EBT scores.

Where it is available: Your physician or local hospital help line should be able to direct you. Most urban areas have EBT availability.

Interpreting the test results: EBT calcium scores range from 0 to over 5,000. The lower the better. A result greater than 1,000 suggests an individual may be in at least the 75th percentile (the high danger zone) for sudden death or a heart attack. The older you get, the more likelihood for calcium deposition to occur as a degenerative process. We normally don't begin to calcify until middle age. It is alarmingly abnormal to encounter a substantial calcium score in a younger person. We would not be concerned with a score of 200 in an eighty-year-old man, but we would be in a forty- or fifty-year-old man. A score of 200 or above in a man under sixty represents a sign of premature aging of the cardiovascular system. Women tend to begin calcifying ten to twenty years later than men. So interpretation of the score has to include gender and age.

When patients come to our office with a calcium score above the 75th percentile, we immediately start testing for markers of inflammation such as CRP and elevated fibrinogen. If test results are positive, that means double trouble—calcified coronary arteries and inflammation. This calls for immediate medical management, including a full diagnostic workup. Speed is of the essence. Knowing your EBT score and then taking action, if necessary, can truly save your life.

We would probably start a patient with a high coronary calcium score and high CRP on a statin drug, not as you might think to lower cholesterol but to take advantage of the drug's anti-inflammatory properties. We would likely prescribe an ACE inhibitor and fish oil. Fish oil is a major weapon because its fatty acid compounds penetrate plaque within three days and help prevent rupture. To help lower CRP, we would also recommend moderate, regular exercise, a daily low-dose aspirin, and antioxidant and mineral supplementation, such as CoQ10 and fish oil.

Carotid Artery Intima Media Thickness

For many years, doctors have put ultrasound devices to good use in helping them diagnose real-time inside-the-body status ranging from fetal development to early prostate cancer. An ultrasound machine transmits sound pulses into the body through a probe. The waves travel into the tissues and encounter various structures and activity. The reflected echoes, captured on imaging screens, enable us to peer inside and witness ongoing activity.

Cardiologists routinely use ultrasound. We check moving blood flow to the heart, look for abnormalities in the function and structure of the organ, and evaluate the heart's ability to deal with the stress of heart failure and recovery from surgery or a heart attack.

Recently, a new ultrasound technique has become available that measures carotid artery intima media thickness (IMT). It is also known as carotid digitally enhanced B-mode ultrasound. The pictures produced of the crucial arteries to the brain provide a reliable, independent risk assessment for both stroke and cardiovascular disease.

The device has a powerful ability to identify soft, noncalcified plaque.

And identifying this life-threatening buildup enables us to better predict who is at risk for serious disease and sudden death. Remember that soft, flexible plaque has a greater tendency to rupture than the solid, calcified (hard) plaque that's picked up through EBT scanning.

Diagnostics have done a good job in readily identifying hard plaques and then bypassing them with surgery. But one of the major shortcomings has been the failure to locate the softer lesions that are prone to rupture.

Doctors prefer to screen their patients as noninvasively as possible before ordering more invasive testing procedures. In that context, IMT has become a cutting-edge noninvasive procedure just as echocardiography was twenty-five years ago.

With IMT we can spot a dangerous, probably widespread risk factor that would otherwise be missed. People with soft plaques in the carotids are likely to have similar plaques in the blood vessels to the heart. Blockages in any part of the circulatory system suggest plaque buildup elsewhere.

The American Heart Association has endorsed this procedure as an effective method of assessing blockages that haven't yet created clinical signs and symptoms. The association has stated that for people without symptoms who are over the age of 45, IMT adds a substantial level of improvement to traditional risk factor assessment. As with the EBT score, the rate of change of the carotid IMT is of greater significance than one single IMT result at a single point in time.

Who should have the test: Consider IMT if you have a strong family history of heart disease or stroke, have multiple cardiovascular risk factors, and/or are ultravigilant about early cardiovascular disease. Often the test is used with Doppler imaging of carotid blood flow to determine whether plaque is causing any disturbance to the brain.

Pros: IMT is a safe and inexpensive technique. The cost is about $180. It is generally covered by insurance.

Where it is available: IMT is usually available in major medical centers and cardiologists' offices.

Interpreting the test results: A therapy program of nutraceutical and pharmaceutical agents can be employed to help reverse the process if soft plaque is found in the carotid arteries, similar to our approach to a markedly abnormal EBT. Here, however, we would lean more toward phosphatidylcholine supplementation to encourage reverse cholesterol transport (more on this in chapter 6).

Chapter 5

Medication

What You Need and Don't Need

Some of the patients who come to our office are zealous believers in alternative medicine, dead-set against medical drugs because of the side effects. They insist on pharmaceutical-free treatment.

We consider ourselves integrative physicians. We use the best of conventional drugs, nutritional supplements, and, when we deem necessary, surgery.

If we personally were to have a heart attack, a bypass, or a stent procedure, we would have no problem taking specific drugs, for instance, a statin or an angiotensin-converting enzyme (ACE) inhibitor. We tell patients what we would do for ourselves and what we would do in their situations. In some cases, we feel comfortable recommending a program based totally on supplements. In other cases, we suggest a combination of supplements and pharmaceuticals because we feel the supplements will achieve a better long-term outcome with specific medical drugs. And sometimes we strongly recommend medication to rescue patients out of immediate crisis, reserving the supplements for a later, safer date when we can begin chipping away at the underlying causes of their problem.

This is the integrative approach. We're not biased against anything. We are for whatever works the best for the individual patient.

Some patients, however, still refuse to take drugs. In such cases, we feel obliged to honor their wishes and come up with an effective supplement plan. Chapters 6 and 7 will cover the most effective supplements for the prevention and stabilization of plaque. In this chapter, we will discuss the characteristics of the medications used by cardiologists and how they may influence arterial inflammation and plaque. We're sharing our understanding of the relevant research along with our own clinical experience.

Statin Drugs:
Upsides and Downsides

When we speak to lay audiences, we receive many questions about the safety and effectiveness of cholesterol-lowering medications. Questions have multiplied recently because constant news about the serious side effects of major drugs are making people increasingly fearful.

Statins sell under a variety of brand names: Mevacor, Lipitor, Pravachol, Zocor, Lescol, and Crestor. Technically, they are HMG-CoA (3-hydroxy-3-methylglutaryl coenzyme A) reductase inhibitors, meaning they reduce the action of the principal enzyme in the liver that produces cholesterol. The targeted medical effect is to decrease LDL cholesterol.

We use statins extensively but selectively in our practices. They have definite therapeutic value, but they also have definite downsides. They are too often inappropriately prescribed by physicians solely preoccupied with cholesterol.

Every cardiologist in the country seems to be writing prescriptions for statins, with no apparent recognition between patients who may benefit from statin drugs and those who could be better served by alternative methods. We believe this is a travesty.

Statins by the Numbers

Approximately 15 to 20 million Americans currently take statin drugs for cholesterol control. It is estimated the number will climb to more than 36 million as doctors begin to prescribe statins not only to lower cholesterol but also for elevated CRP levels.

Statin drugs are blockbuster sellers, surpassing hypertension medications in generating revenues for pharmaceutical manufacturers. In 2003, they earned an estimated $16 billion.

Statins: The Good News

Without doubt, statins protect patients from heart attack and decrease their need for revascularization procedures, definitely improving quality of life. But new research shows that the protective effect goes way beyond cholesterol reduction, and in one 2006 study showed that a statin drug may possibly reverse plaque.

In 2000, doctors at the University of Utah reported a study in which they monitored 1,707 patients undergoing coronary arteriography. Nearly a thousand of them were diagnosed with severe coronary artery disease. During a three-year period, more than a hundred of these patients died. Cholesterol measurements failed to predict their vulnerability, but statin therapy was associated with improved survival, especially in patients with the highest CRP levels. So statins appeared to be working on another level than lowering cholesterol, namely a reduction in inflammation.

In a German study published in 2002, researchers monitored the outcome of 1,616 patients hospitalized with coronary artery disease and chest pain. They found that patients whose statin drugs were discontinued were nearly three times as likely to have a nonfatal heart attack or die, compared with patients who continued to receive statin therapy. The researchers proposed that stopping statins impaired vascular function independent of lipid-lowering effects.

Also in 2002, British doctors revealed the results of the largest-to-date statin analysis: the Heart Protection Study. It involved more than 20,000 people with vascular disease affecting arteries outside the heart area. Statin therapy was found to exert a positive impact across all patient groups: women, the elderly, diabetics, and people with low cholesterol levels. Even in subjects with acceptable LDL levels (less than 100 mg/dl), there was a clear reduction in major cardiovascular events, indicating that risk reduction for CVD is not just the result of statins reducing LDL cholesterol alone. In 2004, a detailed analysis of twenty-five different studies involving 69,510 patients with coronary artery disease found that statin therapy substantially reduced heart attack and mortality rates even when pretreatment LDL levels were as low as 100 mg/dl.

In these and other continuing studies, the evidence clearly points to cardioprotective properties of statins due more to an anti-inflammatory activity than to their cholesterol-lowering effects.

The research has brought out a fascinating and unheralded aspect of statins: their pleiotropic effect, meaning the drugs have beneficial actions above and beyond cholesterol reduction.

Can Crestor Reverse Plaque?

It was with great interest that we read a highly publicized 2006 study appearing in the *Journal of the American Medical Association* claiming plaque reversal for the Goliath of statin drugs—Crestor.

This very same Crestor has been under fire by the consumer group Public Citizen, which contends that this drug has "unique risks" and should not be prescribed, especially at the dose (40 mg a day) used in the study unless smaller doses and other drugs fail to help. The Food and Drug Administration in 2005 required a warning on its label because of potentially serious kidney and musculoskeletal problems.

In this new study, headed by physicians at the Cleveland Clinic and funded by Crestor maker AstraZeneca PLC, two-thirds of the 349 study participants were reported to have had regression of plaque buildups.

For the first time, a drug showed regression of plaque. The researchers based their finding on intracoronary ultrasound, a technique in which a tiny camera is inserted into the coronary artery. With this technology one can literally scan the inside of the artery and see the plaque load inside the vessel and determine whether there is buildup or regression. However, using this or any ultrasound method always raises the possibility of observer error because it is up to the observer to interpret the visualization of the plaque.

In this study, ultrasound measurements were made before and two years after the start of Crestor treatment. The researchers reported a modest 1 percent reduction of each patient's major blockage. That may not sound like much, but mathematically plaque needs only to shrink a miniscule amount—just a small improvement to the diameter of a blood vessel—to significantly enhance blood flow.

Based on this study, Crestor may be a reasonable choice for symptomatic people with advanced coronary disease who have no other good options—people who are totally clogged, have been bypassed, stented, and rebypassed, and with very high total calcified plaque burdens showing on electron beam tomography.

However, Crestor is reasonable only if patients are protected with at least 200 mg daily of CoQ10 (see chapter 7). That's because statin drugs deplete CoQ10, and Crestor is the most potent statin. Whenever we prescribe less powerful statins, such as Lipitor, we prescribe at least 100 mg daily of CoQ10.

A positive study such as this one often inspires a rush to prescribe. But prescribing Crestor to a forty-year-old with high cholesterol is not smart medicine. It could, in fact, be deadly. It may be valuable for an older (sixty to eighty) patient who can't get another bypass and who has a totally unsatisfactory quality of life, and with the drug he or she can get some plaque regression, symptom improvement, and life extension. That's smarter medicine and where Crestor may be beneficial. As long as the patient can tolerate the drug, then it's worth the risk.

The researchers in the study attributed the good results to Crestor's ability to lower LDL cholesterol. We're not so sure about that conclusion. To us, too low LDL is a double-edged sword. Clinically, we have seen too many people with rock-bottom LDL develop memory problems. LDL may protect you from many toxins, including mercury. LDL also carries CoQ10. You need LDL. We don't want to destroy something that was built into our bodies. There could be other reasons why Crestor is working. One is that it is a potent anti-inflammatory. Another is that it increased HDL cholesterol, the good cholesterol, by 14 percent. Those two effects are more important to us than simply lowering cholesterol. In any case, the result was intriguing, and we look forward to larger follow-up studies.

For one, statins can have a nitric oxide sparing effect that contributes to improved endothelial function of blood vessels. Nitric oxide, a substance produced in the endothelium, promotes healthy dilation of the arteries and inhibits abnormal platelet clotting.

Second, atherosclerotic plaques are under siege from an onslaught of free radicals and inflammatory molecules that can cause a weakening of the fibrous cap, thus making the plaque vulnerable to rupture and placing the individual at immediate risk for heart attack or stroke. Statins increase plaque stability through a variety of mechanisms, including the increase of collagen (structural protein) content in the plaque matrix and suppression of macrophage growth. They have significant anti-inflammatory and antiproliferative effects. It turns out that before they block cholesterol, statins block cellular signaling factors in the body that lead to the production of destructive free radicals and inflammation.

These shotgun properties can also reduce the threat of stroke. Statins can stabilize plaque in the carotid artery as well as in the aortic arch, the first large artery receiving blood when the heart contracts. This is why we use statins in patients with advanced plaque of the carotids and high EBT calcium scores.

Who Should and Should Not Take Statins

We have little doubt that statin therapy cuts the incidence of heart disease, especially for those at the greatest risk. Patients with the most to gain and the least to lose are men, aged forty-five to sixty-five, with proven coronary artery disease.

As a general rule, it makes sense to consider statin therapy in patients with:

- A history of blocked coronary arteries, heart attack, TIA, or stroke
- Prior stent implantation, bypass, or angioplasty
- Diabetes, a high CRP level, and other risk factors but no heart disease
- A high coronary calcium score on EBT (see EBT discussion in chapter 4), especially in the presence of inflammatory markers such as high CRP and fibrinogen

In our opinion, statins aren't indicated for generally healthy people with:

- No history or evidence of vascular disease
- No history of previous heart attacks
- Normal CRP level (less than 1 mg/L)
- Zero or low (less than 200) EBT score

We don't prescribe statin drugs to lower cholesterol. We selectively use statins to improve outcome in patients with risk markers known to respond well to this drug intervention.

Although more study is needed, the same pleiotropic activities may make statins appropriate for some heart valve conditions. Consider calcific aortic stenosis, a problem frequently seen by cardiologists. For years we thought that calcific deposition inside cardiac valves was due to gradual wear and tear accompanying the aging process. Now we know that there may be an active inflammatory process at work in the delicate valvular structures. Valve replacement was once the only option we could offer patients. Now we have statins. They decrease blood cell adhesiveness and plaque calcification, important characteristics of calcific aortic valvular disease. Statins have other beneficial effects:

- They may cut the risk of bone fracture. In four large studies, the risk of hip and nonspinal fractures was considerably reduced among patients taking statins. Animal experiments have demonstrated that statins increase bone formation in rodents, suggesting the drugs may be useful in the treatment of osteoporosis.

- Multiple sclerosis (MS) patients may benefit. MS is an autoimmune disorder that destroys myelin, the fatty sheath around nerve cells. In animal studies, statins reversed paralysis in mice with MS and prevented a relapse of the disease. It's not known exactly how statins work in this regard. A large controlled trial is now under way.

- Statins may improve macular degeneration, an age-related disorder in which cholesterol accumulates in membranes of the eye.

- Trials are now under way to clarify a potential role in cancer. So far results are mixed. Statins have improved prostate and bowel cancers and acute myeloid leukemia, but in Japan there was an increase in lymphomas in patients taking very strong statins. It may take much more research to figure this out.

- Some research data suggest that statins may prevent a buildup of beta-amyloid in the brain, thus delaying the onset of Alzheimer's disease. This protein is associated with senile plaques that are involved in the disruption of thinking. Clinical trials are under way.

Statins: The Bad News

The research looks promising. But what about side effects? Remember that pharmaceutical therapy, even when appropriately applied, remains the fourth leading cause of death in the United States.

We see a big problem brewing because of the common practice of prescribing statins to healthy individuals with no history or evidence of arterial disease. In our opinion, doctors who prescribe these drugs for high cholesterol levels alone, in the absence of previous coronary disease, diabetes, or high CRP, do not practice good medicine. The overuse of these potent pharmacological agents with known and unknown side effects as a long-term strategy in otherwise healthy people is risky business and simply not justified. Long-term risk assessments are not known.

As practicing cardiologists, we can personally attest to numerous side effects that go beyond what is generally reported. We have heard a lot of colleagues say that the muscle pain you hear about just doesn't exist. Our response: either they don't see enough patients or they don't ask the right questions. One-third of the patients we see can't take statin medications.

The common side effects: muscle pain and weakness, flulike symptoms, and soreness. In severe cases, muscle cells can break down (rhabdomyolysis) and release myoglobin into the blood, an iron-containing protein pigment similar to hemoglobin. Too much myoglobin impairs the kidneys, leading to kidney failure and even death. Other side effects include liver dysfunction with elevation of liver enzymes, a nervous system disorder called polyneuropathy, and total global amnesia in which patients forget where and who they are for a few minutes to several hours at a time. If the LDL level drops too low, it can interfere with neurotransmitter mechanisms in the brain.

Statins predispose you to heart failure. It takes energy for the heart muscle to relax, just as it takes energy for it to contract and pump out blood. This nonstop operation depends on adequate ATP, the fuel of cellular bioenergetics. Your heart cells, as well as all other cells in your body, need CoQ10 to produce adequate ATP. Statins block the formation of CoQ10. They interfere with a biochemical pathway shared by both cholesterol and CoQ10.

With less ATP to meet the heart's enormous energy demands, the organ becomes stiff. It can't relax. Blood pressure within the heart rises. The increased pressure transmits back to the lungs, and patients may experience shortness of breath, initially with exertion and later even at rest if the process continues unchecked. All patients with heart failure have abnormal heart stiffness known as diastolic dysfunction. It is the sole cause of heart failure in some. A study published in the *American Journal of Cardiology* demonstrated that statin therapy can produce diastolic dysfunction in subjects initially free of heart failure. In patients with poor cardiac pump function, statin therapy can reduce the function further and generate outright heart failure. This was first reported in 1990 and again in 2004. Some clinicians believe that widespread statin use has contributed to the soaring incidence of heart failure in the United States.

The pharmaceutical industry likes to claim that statin drugs save lives. Indeed, large studies carried out in patients with known CVD have consistently shown a reduction in cardiac events and death rates with statin therapy as compared to placebo. We agree with these conclusions. However, the studies also consistently tell us that cholesterol lowering is associated with an increased death rate due to other causes, such as cancer, suicide, and motor vehicle accidents. Why this rise in disparate deaths? Researchers haven't given us the precise answers yet. Perhaps when LDL becomes too low it cannot perform its tasks in the body, one of which is

Stiff Hearts: A Statin Side Effect

In New Cardiology, the heart is all about energy—keeping the living pump working and improving its filling power. Most cardiologists concern themselves primarily with the contraction of the heart, the systolic phase of pumping out the blood. But we also pay a lot of attention to the diastolic phase—filling the heart with blood—because that activity requires more energy.

Without enough energy, your heart fibers get stuck and stiffen up. You get a stiff heart that can't relax. Doctors call this diastolic dysfunction. Half of heart failures occur because the heart can't relax. This is where the ATP comes in. It takes more ATP to relax the heart after contraction.

This stiffness phenomenon is insidious. The problem brews for years. At first there are no signs of trouble. Then one day you notice something isn't right. You go to your doctor and complain about getting fatigued more or experiencing shortness of breath. You can't understand why.

The doctor checks you out, does an echocardiogram showing a normal systolic function and a normal ejection fraction (the measurement of the contraction force that pumps the blood out into the body). The doctor may say that everything is okay and that you need to relax more.

This is an important issue. Mitral valve prolapse, for instance, is all about diastolic dysfunction and energy deficit. A lot of people have it, particularly women. Their heart can't fill with blood adequately. They get more diastolic dysfunction from high blood pressure and thus suffer more as a result than men with high blood pressure.

No drugs can help with diastolic dysfunction. Only CoQ10, D-ribose, carnitine, and magnesium supplementation improve this dysfunction in our experience.

---

to help detoxify harmful substances such as mercury. But the facts are disturbing and question the growing practice of putting young people without CVD on statins for the purpose of prevention.

Another point: statin drugs are expensive. They cost around $100 a month. If your risk is low, say 2 chances out of 100 that you will sustain a CVD event, and statin therapy reduces your risk to 1 chance out of 100 (the 50 percent risk reduction rate the drug companies talk about), should you spend $1,200 per year for the rest of your life to take a drug that will not prolong your life? Vitamin C delays the rate at which arteries clog, decreases cardiovascular event rate, and lowers overall mortality. Vitamin

C costs pennies a day. Antioxidants and essential fatty acids do the same for $250 a year.

The big fallout from statin abuse is coming. We track the research carefully. We take care of thousands of patients. We ourselves would be the first to take a statin if we had high coronary calcification, particularly in the critical left main coronary artery, or a stent, or a bypass, or a previous heart attack. We want the drug for its high-powered anti-inflammatory effect in those threatening situations. But we would also take a high dose of CoQ10 with it because we know that statins deplete CoQ10 in the body. Some researchers have described heart failure as primarily a CoQ10 deficiency disease. A lower CoQ10 level has also been cited as a contributing factor in breast cancer—a finding that should be a cause for caution when prescribing statins to postmenopausal women, a high-risk population for breast cancer.

The bottom line is that statins can work for you or against you. Everyone is unique and has to weigh the potential risk/reward ratio. If you have a family history of high lipids, early heart attacks, and premature death, you may opt to be more aggressive.

But suppose you are a young male or female in your forties with no history of heart disease. Your laboratory evaluation reveals normal blood sugar, low CRP, and elevated cholesterol. Your physician wants to prescribe a statin to lower your cholesterol. If it works, he or she will keep you on it for the rest of your life. Should you go for it? This scenario weighs heavy on the risk side and light on the benefit side.

Remember that cholesterol does not accurately predict heart disease. We regard it as a national tragedy that millions of young people without any of the risk factors go on statins. They have the least to gain and the most to lose.

Coumadin

Over the years, hundreds of patients have approached us wanting to discontinue their Coumadin prescription. They're tired of the frequent blood draws necessary to monitor the anticoagulant effect and they're worried about the risk of abnormal bleeding. These issues, in fact, are major reasons why patients come to see us in the first place.

Warfarin (more commonly known by its brand name Coumadin) is widely used in cardiology to prevent blood clots from forming or growing larger. We prescribe it for certain types of irregular heartbeat, when ultrasound determines a thrombus (clot) in the heart, and following placement of a mechanical heart valve.

Coumadin blocks the action of vitamin K, the body's naturally occurring fat-soluble vitamin essential for blood clotting. Vitamin K contributes to the production of a protein in the liver involved in the clotting process.

In chapter 6, we will discuss the alternatives to Coumadin, such as the natural clot busters nattokinase and lumbrokinase. But at this time we do not recommend them for patients highly vulnerable to clot formation or stroke related to clot dislodgement, where Coumadin has a long track record of protection. The alternatives are fine if we are treating young patients with normal functioning valves and no heart chamber enlargement.

Doctors prescribing Coumadin to patients periodically check on the drug's activity in the body through a blood test called Protime or PT/INR (short for prothrombin time/international normalization ratio). The test assesses the amount of time it takes for blood to form clots. The results help doctors determine the safest and most effective dosage. If you take Coumadin, be sure to have your level checked according to your doctor's instructions.

Doctors prescribing Coumadin will sometimes tell their patients not to take any vitamins. We disagree. Vitamins are simply too important for health maintenance and healing to simply discard, especially for chronically ill patients in need of extra nutritional support.

The Vitamin K Issue

One of the most damaging myths has been perpetuated by doctors who tell patients on Coumadin to avoid foods rich in vitamin K such as green leafy vegetables, radishes, cabbage, broccoli, spinach, kale, beans, and asparagus. Their reasoning: they interfere with the effectiveness of the medication. Doctors may also say not to take supplements with vitamin K (they usually come in multivitamin formulas).

Our concern: the body needs vitamin K for bone strength and for the integrity of arteries, including the coronary blood vessels in the heart. A deficiency leads to weak bones and hip fractures. Moreover, a series of recent studies has pointed to poor vitamin K status as a significant risk factor for severe coronary artery calcification.

The dilemma we face is that Coumadin is a vitamin K antagonist, and when vitamin K levels fall, the propensity for arterial damage increases.

Obviously, we don't want this to happen to our patients. Thus, we are concerned about the long-term use of Coumadin, especially since doctors usually tell patients to take the medication for the rest of their lives. We believe that our patients should protect themselves by getting enough vitamin K in their diet.

If you include vitamin K foods in your diet and you are on Coumadin, just try to maintain a steady intake of those particular foods. Routine monitoring of your PT/INR value will ensure that you are getting an effective dosage of medication. Adjustments can be made if necessary.

Beware: Coumadin Interactions

Fish oil. Keep the level of fish oil to about 3 grams or less if you take Coumadin. Greater than 6 grams a day has been shown to increase bleeding vulnerability.

Garlic. Avoid garlic supplementation if you take Coumadin. The blood-thinning properties of both can make the blood too thin.

Ginkgo biloba. Ginkgo inhibits clotting activity to some degree. Thus, to avoid excessive bleeding, don't take it with Coumadin or any other anti-platelet agents.

Saint-John's-wort. This popular herb may weaken the therapeutic effect of Coumadin by promoting certain liver enzymes to clear medication from the body faster. Don't take it with Coumadin.

Other medications. Many medications impair or intensify the effectiveness of Coumadin. Whenever you change your regimen, get a repeat blood check. Ask your physician about a possible interaction.

Angiotensin-Converting Enzyme Inhibitors

Angiotensin-converting enzyme (ACE) is a potent agent produced in the lungs that converts angiotensin I, a harmless molecule, into angiotensin II, the most potent blood vessel constrictor known to science. ACE-inhibiting drugs, used for more than twenty-five years in the treatment of high blood pressure, slow down ACE activity, resulting in relaxation of blood vessel walls, lower blood pressure, and a reduced burden on the heart.

When we look at all the factors that activate and inflame artery wall tissue, we find ACE right up there among them. The enzyme stimulates adhesion molecules and oxidative stress. It also depletes the body of zinc and may interact negatively with L-arginine, the amino acid that feeds the production of nitric oxide in endothelial cells. Nitric oxide keeps arteries dilated. ACE inhibitors block the formation of free radicals and preserve nitric oxide.

ACE is pathologically overactive in atherosclerosis. For instance, someone with unstable angina has ten times more of it in plaque than someone with stable angina. The enzyme contributes to vulnerability in plaque because it produces free radical stress and inflammation, fanning the process that weakens the fibrous envelope of the plaque, allowing the witches' brew inside to leak out.

Some of the leading ACE medications include Capoten, Altace, Accupril, Lotensin, and Prinivil. Not all ACE inhibitors are the same. We prefer the fat-soluble drugs such as Altace and Accupril that are tissue specific—that is, they work both in the circulation and in the endothelium to block free radical activity and in the process improve nitric oxide production. The first ACE inhibitors, such as Capoten, work only in the circulation. They are fine for high blood pressure and heart failure, but they do not discourage vascular inflammation.

We see better results with the tissue-specific inhibitors that work both in the blood and in the cells. They help prevent restenosis after stent implantation and improve outcome after open heart surgery. They decrease future adverse event rates in diabetics.

Who should use a tissue-specific ACE inhibitor? It's a standard prescriptive drug for high blood pressure that has additional benefits. We recommend it for patients with symptomatic atherosclerosis, plaque, or who have had heart attacks. Heart attacks damage and weaken some of the heart muscle, making it more difficult for the heart to pump blood. ACE inhibitors can be utilized after a cardiac event to keep arteries relaxed and maximally open so that more blood can reach the heart muscle.

High blood pressure in the presence of a high calcium score (determined by EBT testing) and an abundance of plaque increases the danger of plaque rupture. The rational pharmaceutical approach to stabilize and perhaps reverse this situation is to use an ACE inhibitor such as Altace or Accupril in combination with a statin.

We would first strive to improve endothelial health with supplements rather than with ACE inhibitors. However, ACE inhibitors have a positive benefit-to-risk ratio and will result in fewer cardiovascular emergencies. These drugs are good choices by your doctor.

The major downside is a nonthreatening and annoying dry cough, and it happens fairly frequently. It is what makes some people want to stop the drug.

Angiotensin Receptor Blockers

If a patient complains about the cough while taking an ACE inhibitor, we would switch him or her to an angiotensin receptor blocker (ARB). ACE inhibitors slow down the production of angiotensin II. ARBs lock into the cell membrane binding sites of angiotensin II and basically block its influence on cell biochemistry. The action is similar to Tamoxifen, which blocks cellular binding sites in the body for estrogen.

ARBs appear to help in heart failure and kidney disease, but we haven't seen any research showing significant benefit for coronary artery disease.

Beta Blockers

For patients with coronary artery disease or heart failure, beta blockers can be lifesavers. They are among the most effective and safest drugs we have in cardiology.

These medications block the beta sympathetic limb of the autonomic nervous system, the part responsible for gearing up your body for action. Beta blockers lower blood pressure, relieve angina, and help prevent further ischemic damage in heart attack patients. They decrease the heart's need for blood and oxygen by reducing its workload. They also help the heart to beat more regularly and discourage surges in heart rate and blood pressure in times of stress. Beta blockers and ACE inhibitors decrease the risk of adverse cardiovascular events well beyond what would be expected from blood pressure reduction alone.

Research tells us that individuals who take beta blockers for a year after a heart attack have a lower incidence of sudden cardiac death and recurrent heart attacks. Some doctors use beta blockers after a heart attack to stabilize arrhythmia. Our feeling is that beta blockers will also help stabilize vulnerable plaque in patients with angina and hypertension who may be subject to adrenaline surges from anger, panic, and stress. More research is needed in this area. Nevertheless, a beta blocker is a good drug for stressed, hypertensive individuals.

Beta blockers are sometimes used by actors to prevent stage fright caused by anxiety. We have prescribed them to professional golfers to steady their hands while putting. They can calm down the body's response to threat, uncertainty, and fear.

As with all drugs, there are some downsides. We don't like to use beta blockers for elderly patients because they might cause mental confusion. There are different types of beta blockers available that you can talk to your doctor about. When appropriate, the medication should be of the cardio-selective type.

Standard, non-cardio-selective beta blockers can trigger asthma attacks. If you have asthma and take one of the standard medications, you could get worse. In heart failure, Coreg is the drug of choice if you don't mind spending an extra $100 a month. It also functions as an antioxidant. Insurance often covers this medication but not always. Some people may not tolerate Coreg, but most do. Benefits may not be experienced for months.

These drugs have the potential to amplify depressive symptoms in people already depressed. Other possible side effects include nightmares, diarrhea, and erectile dysfunction. But for a vulnerable patient after a heart attack with advanced plaque and high blood pressure, a beta blocker is a good choice.

Calcium Blockers

Doctors use this class of antihypertensive drugs to reduce the tone of the arterial wall, aiming to improve blood flow through narrowed vessels. Although calcium blockers are effective for high blood pressure, they have a destabilizing influence on heart rate variability. Their long-term record is troubling. In an overview of nine large-scale clinical trials, the drugs were associated with 25 percent higher rates of both acute heart attacks and heart failure compared to other types of medication.

If you had a heart attack and take these drugs that affect the variable rate of the heart, there could be disastrous consequences. As a general rule, we don't prescribe calcium blockers or alpha blockers, drugs used for prostate disease that also negatively impact heart rate variability.

Moreover, calcium blockers cause ankle swelling. When that occurs, a doctor often prescribes a diuretic. Then the patient needs to take potassium. A whole new side disease has essentially been created. Calcium blockers are drugs of last resort. Supplemental magnesium does what calcium blockers can do, and more, but without the risks.

Aspirin

Some cardiologists recommend that everyone over age forty take a daily low-dose aspirin as part of good cardiovascular prevention. Aspirin can help keep your blood thinner.

We don't make this recommendation to healthy people for primary CVD prevention. The reason: aspirin may seem harmless, but it's one of the leading causes of gastrointestinal bleeding.

We prefer a variety of supplements that keep the blood at a healthy viscosity without eroding the digestive tract. They include fish oil, garlic, ginger, bromelain, full-spectrum vitamin E (with both alpha and gamma tocopherol), and magnesium.

Painkillers and Heart Disease

Revelations in 2004 and 2005 that best-selling painkillers such as Vioxx, Celebrex, Aleve, and Bextra increase the risk of heart attacks made big headlines. The news stunned millions of patients relying on these medications. Ongoing news about possible adverse cardiovascular effects from medication makes us very concerned about the widespread use of painkillers altogether.

They all, in fact, have side effects, even over-the-counter pharmaceuticals such as acetaminophen (liver-related problems) and nonsteroidal anti-inflammatories (NSAIDs) such as ibuprofen (high blood pressure and weakened kidneys). Prescription NSAIDs are even stronger. Overuse of NSAIDs has ruined the careers and health of several well-known professional athletes. If NSAIDs can harm young people in peak physical shape, think of what they can do to you.

Recent research shows that NSAIDs can hamper the mitochondrial production of adenosine triphosphate (ATP), the body's basic cellular fuel. In essence, many of these analgesics act like mitochondrial toxins.

ATP is vital to the proper functioning of all cells and particularly to the cells of the heart muscle that pump nonstop. When drugs curtail this energy production, something has to give.

Cardiologists are caught in a dilemma of what's best for a heart patient with severe arthritis when perhaps the only medication that helps the pain is an anti-inflammatory. Should the patient take it and be active or not take it and become a couch potato?

Our approach to people with chronic arthritic pain is to recommend natural anti-inflammatories such as fish oil, glucosamine, chondroitin, MSM, and willow bark. For now, we don't recommend the pharmaceutical anti-inflammatory drugs because they have too many downsides. In any case, two of the leading products—Vioxx and Bextra—have already been withdrawn from the market, and manufacturers of many other popular drugs in this class, both prescription and over-the-counter products, have been told by the FDA to include label warnings about potential health risks.

Chapter 6

Supplements

The Basics

Most doctors today prescribe drugs for specific effects such as lowering cholesterol or blood pressure. When the drugs don't work, surgeons may be called in to perform lifesaving bypasses or heart transplants. In integrative medicine, we use or recommend these approaches as well. But we have learned to do something extra, something normally ignored, absolutely simplistic, and bargain-basement cheap compared to dazzling, big-ticket technology. We optimize nutritional status—with vitamins, minerals, antioxidants, and other natural substances—to help the body heal itself.

Before 1990, vitamins and minerals were seen by most physicians as substances in food that prevented nutritional deficiency states such as scurvy, beriberi, rickets, and pellagra. Mainstream medicine viewed supplementation as unnecessary, believing people got all the nutrition they needed from their diet. For decades, only a small minority of nutritionally oriented physicians recommended supplements as a potent, safe, and inexpensive medical option . . . and many of them actually got in trouble for doing that.

Today we realize that vast numbers of people eat poorly and do not get the proper nutrition from their diets that their bodies need to sustain good health. Moreover, a global wave of positive nutritional research has rendered the conventional viewpoint on supplementation utterly obsolete. Many thousands of published studies have shown that individual nutrients at doses higher than those usually present in food have a significant preventive and therapeutic effect for serious diseases, not just nutritional deficiency states.

In 2002, the standard-bearer for mainstream U.S. medicine, the *Journal of the American Medical Association*, published a report from Harvard researchers acknowledging that "most people do not consume an optimal amount of all vitamins by diet alone." Because of this suboptimal intake and the "strong evidence of effectiveness" from controlled trials, "it appears prudent for all adults to take vitamin supplements."

The wealth of research has greatly influenced the way the two of us practice cardiology. Unlike most cardiologists, a comprehensive supplement program is a major part of our practice. The supplements address specific cardiovascular shortcomings and simultaneously strengthen overall physiology to fight off infection, inflammation, and plaque, nourish the nervous and endocrine systems, and give extra oomph to the whole body.

Sick people need this nutritional upgrade . . . and they benefit magnificently. It often keeps them out of the hospital. Sometimes the supplements work rapidly like magic. Patients suddenly become rejuvenated as their nutritionally starved bodies respond to healing nutrients missing for years. Other times we see a steady but remarkable return to health by patients who previously sputtered along on near-empty tanks. Now, with their tanks full, they move actively forward in life, feeling better than they have in years.

Supplement Teamwork: A Misunderstood Principle

Used alone, single nutritional supplements can often generate powerful effects in the body. We strongly believe, however, they work best in combination—as a team—rather than just one or two alone. As an example, we can best combat the oxidative damage from free radicals with a combination of antioxidants, each packing different strengths and abilities. Vitamins C, E, CoQ10, bioflavonoids, alpha-lipoic acid, beta-carotene, lycopene, and selenium are a few of the important antioxidants. Having just one working for you—like vitamin C—but none of the others is like fielding a team with one all-star and no supporting players. We want the whole team in action, not one player alone.

Dr. Roberts: Years ago, as a busy cardiologist in my midthirties, I believed that vitamin therapy was bogus medicine with the potential to harm patients. I believed this because my professors had told me so. There was no scientific backing for this teaching, just bias, ignorance, and blind allegiance to the glories of a pharmaceutical and surgical paradigm. Of course, the fact that the pharmaceutical industry funds our journals, our meetings, and a good deal of medical school activities and research also helps explain the attitude. And I, like my hardworking peers, was totally sold out to a drug and invasive treatment approach to CVD.

One day, a persistent patient—a retired army colonel—who was tired of repeated treatments without getting better, pressed a research paper into my hand. It discussed the benefits of antioxidant vitamins for cardiac patients. He dogged me until I finally read the paper.

The research made sense. It talked about how antioxidants actually addressed the underlying cause of his blocked arteries. It may sound strange at this point in time, but for a superachieving crisis doctor the concept of treating the causes of cardiovascular disease, not just the consequences, was pretty alien.

I began reading up on nutritional medicine and started recommending supplements to my patients. Soon I had nearly all of my patients taking multivitamins. As I learned about other healing nutrients, I prescribed vitamins more and more.

My hospital admitting rate fell like a rock. In time, I was seeing my patients for checkups and tune-ups in the office as opposed to repeated crisis intervention in the hospital.

I'm still doing heart catheterizations, and my patients undergo angioplasty, stent placement, and bypass surgery if I think they need it, but these patients, just like all my patients, are also treated nutritionally, and they do much better. This is incredibly gratifying to me.

Vitamin C can neutralize some free radicals, but alone it has no effect on many others. It can also be consumed in the battle against free radicals. Spent vitamin C, however, can be recharged by bioflavonoids (vitamin P) if these substances are present in the body. Bioflavonoids are found in citrus fruit and vegetables, as well as in supplemental form. Vitamin C and bioflavonoids can be purchased in combined formulations.

In turn, vitamin C recharges spent vitamin E. And vitamin E works within cells with lycopene, beta-carotene, and CoQ10, antioxidants that target different free radicals.

Nature expects us to take in hundreds of nutrients each day to support the body's constant health protection and healing operations. And that's where nutritional supplements can make a big contribution, above and beyond eating a variety of wholesome foods.

Some of the individual supplements we recommend may be part of a multiple nutrient formulation. Others are needed in larger individual quantities than what may be contained in the multiple. You can buy most of these supplements in health food stores. If you can't, we'll let you know where you can get them.

This principle of team nutritional medicine makes perfect sense, but for many it takes a long time to understand. Unfortunately, many researchers and health care providers still don't get it. And the consumers are left totally confused by a barrage of conflicting media reports that give shallow information based on flawed studies.

As an example, take a Finnish study covered widely in the press a few years ago. In this particular experiment, longtime middle-aged smokers received either a harmless placebo or 50 international units (IU) of synthetic vitamin E every day for six years. At the end of the study, the researchers found no difference in cardiac events or lung cancer rates between the vitamin E and placebo groups. The researchers did not conclude that the vitamin didn't work, only that at this dosage in smokers it had no effect on new-onset cardiovascular disease and lung cancer. Yet evening news reports said that vitamin E was no more effective than placebo. Doctors used this study to discourage the use of vitamin E by their patients.

Smoking depletes vitamin E in the body. Smoking also destroys vitamin C that is absolutely fundamental to the health of your arterial and immune systems. The Finnish study did not include vitamin C, so the subjects remained C deficient throughout. Finns drink a lot, and alcohol blocks vitamin E absorption from food. They are also notoriously deficient in selenium, without which all the vitamin E in the world cannot protect you, and also in essential fatty acids, a major element in cardiac protection.

So giving these nutritionally deficient, habitual smokers 50 IU of a synthetic and incomplete form of vitamin E and expecting a six-year health benefit is like giving a glass of water to a person dying of thirst in the middle of the Sahara. Even if the smokers had been given 1,000 IU of vitamin E a day, it still might not have worked.

Compared to the Finnish study, a 2004 experiment with Japanese smokers was better designed and demonstrated the importance of applying antioxidants as a team. Researchers from the National Defense Medical College gave fifteen healthy young male smokers both vitamin E and vitamin C for just under a month. The investigators wanted to see how the vitamins would affect the ability of endothelial cells to produce nitric oxide for normal arterial dilation. Their conclusion: oral antioxidant supplements significantly restored function in smokers' damaged arteries. As this and many other studies are proving, supplement combinations have enhanced effects. Here are some outstanding examples:

- Vitamin C or E alone decreases three-year carotid artery disease progression by 5 percent, but taken together, progression is slowed down 45 percent.

- A "cocktail" of vitamins C, F, A, and beta-carotene improves post–heart attack recovery and decreases the death rate by one-third in the critical one-month aftermath.

- Antioxidant combinations protect against arrhythmia and heart attack in patients undergoing bypass surgery.

- Vitamins C and E together versus either one alone work better in preventing disease progression in men following bypass surgery.

- Antioxidant combinations decrease plaque buildup in the arteries of patients receiving heart transplants.

In this chapter, we will spotlight some of the most important supplements that we find to be very effective for CVD prevention as well as specifically address inflammation, plaque stabilization, plaque reversal, and heart failure. There are too many supplements to cover all of them. In chapter 7, we cover three additional supplements—CoQ10, L-carnitine, and D-ribose—that serve as powerful cardiac energizers. In chapter 12, we put our recommendations together and suggest what to take, how much, and when.

Multivitamin/Mineral with Antioxidants

First and foremost, as a foundation for any supplement program, you need a broad-spectrum "multi"—capsules or tablets packed with combinations of vitamins, minerals, antioxidants, and other nutritional factors. Unfortunately, the really good formulas with potent amounts of therapeutically important substances cannot be crammed into a single pill. Usually, a daily serving involves two, three, or more pills. Our patients take multiformulas that consist of up to eight pills twice a day.

Many patients complain about taking a lot of pills—whether supplements or medication. That's understandable. But a one-a-day supplement doesn't cut it—too much is missing. The typical one-a-day multivitamins, such as those advertised on TV, provide little protection. They lack both potency and many of the new-generation antioxidants found in the better formulations sold in health food stores. The better combinations give you healing amounts of B vitamins, magnesium, bioflavonoids, lycopene, lutein, and other supportive nutrients for the cardiovascular system. Moreover, they are made to be more absorbable. You pay more, but you get more. We like multivitamins that are low in beta-carotene (less than 10,000 IU per day), do not contain iron, and offer a variety of vitamin E compounds (see vitamin E discussion further on in this chapter).

Most medical studies on supplements involve single nutrients. Very few consider multiple vitamin formulas because they have such diverse ingredients and potencies. Two studies on multivitamins have impressed us: one in Sweden, reported in the *Journal of Nutrition* in 2003, and the other in the *Canadian Journal of Cardiology* in 1996. Both made similar conclusions: multiple vitamins substantially lower the risk of cardiovascular disease.

No two multiformulas are alike. Products contain some similar basic ingredients but vary widely thereafter. They all have differences in quality, forms of specific nutrients, and potencies. The percentages shown on the labels refer to the National Academy of Science's current RDAs—the recommended daily allowances of essential nutrients thought to be adequate to meet the nutritional needs of healthy people. These values constantly change as a result of ongoing research. Academy experts themselves acknowledge the values to be far from precise. Moreover, the requirements for many nutrients have not been established and in all likelihood other essential nutrients will be found in years to come. There are no official guidelines covering intake for unhealthy individuals.

Fish Oil

Like any machine, your heart needs oil to run smoothly. Not just any oil. Scientific research has identified the right oil as omega-3 fatty acids, oily substances present in plants and fish. We all have a particularly big need for these substances because of unhealthy dietary trends over the years.

One way to get them into your body is to eat a lot of fish. Another way is to take omega-3 fatty acid supplements derived from fish oil. Flaxseed oil supplements came along in recent years as an alternative, a plant source of omega-3s. But, like other omega-3s extracted from plant oils, flaxseed has a short shelf life and is prone to oxidation and rancidity. It requires refrigeration to protect it from becoming rancid. Our preference is fish oil.

Fish oil contains eicosapentaenoic acid (EPA) and docosahexaenoic acid (DHA), highly beneficial compounds for the body. Normally, the human liver must convert omega-3s from plant sources into EPA and DHA. The conversion requires a great deal of energy as well as the presence of a specific enzyme (delta-6-desaturase) that is lacking in some people. Thus, consuming omega-3s in the form of DHA and EPA from fish or fish oil supplements is a much more efficient way of supplying the body.

Beginning in the mid-1970s, Danish investigators discovered that Greenland Eskimos had a low incidence of heart attacks compared to Westerners. The researchers attributed the hardiness of Eskimo hearts to a diet with abundant fish oil, which they felt had potential antiatherosclerotic benefits.

This original study inspired more than forty-five hundred scientific investigations of omega-3 fatty acids on metabolism and health and resulted in repeated confirmation of cardiovascular benefits. For instance, the same low heart attack incidence was found among Japanese, who also ate a diet rich in fish oil.

In 2000, the strength of research prompted the U.S. Food and Drug Administration (FDA) to authorize limited supplement claims about the cardiovascular benefits of EPA and DHA fatty acids. Specifically, labels could mention "supportive evidence" that omega-3s may reduce the risk of coronary artery disease. The FDA oversees nutritional and medication label claims, and does not easily grant such permission for supplements. In 2004, a similar qualified claim was permitted for fish.

Based on the medical research and personal validation from our own clinical experience, fish oil supplements should be part of all cardiovascular treatment programs. Fish oil obtained directly from eating fish or from taking supplements decreases your risk of developing CVD and plaque. If you have plaque, it slows the rate at which plaque advances and protects against plaque rupture, thus decreasing the risk of heart attack, sudden death, atrial fibrillation, or arrhythmia.

Every cardiologist should be interested in the following benefits of fish oil:

- Decreases Lp(a), triglycerides, and blood pressure
- Increases HDL
- Reduces arterial wall inflammation
- Improves endothelial function
- Makes blood less stickier and less likely to form clots
- Stabilizes and maybe even reverses plaque, and prevents plaque rupture
- Soothes heart rate variability, which counteracts arrhythmias
- Contributes to the bioenergy of the heart muscle

Fish oil helps control eicosanoids, tiny, hormonelike substances produced by all your cells. These chemicals have a regulatory influence on inflammatory and immune responses, the integrity of blood vessels, and much, much more. Just like cholesterol, some eicosanoids are considered good and others bad.

The good news: you exert a good deal of control over eicosanoids by what you eat. Foods such as partially hydrogenated fats (trans fats) and refined carbohydrates trigger the production of harmful eicosanoids and promote inflammation. Adequate omega-3 fatty acids prevent and counteract inflammation. Omega-3s benefit just about every tissue in the body.

Fish oil is preventive and therapeutic for all arrhythmias. Atrial fibrillation patients on fish oil are more likely to maintain good heart rhythm. Patients taking fish oil leave the hospital sooner following bypass surgery and are at reduced risk for bypass graft closure. They can walk farther on a treadmill test. And those who are taking nitroglycerin need less of it.

We have prescribed fish oil aggressively to patients for more than a decade. Every patient with plaque gets fish oil. They do better. And it is an incredibly nontoxic substance.

Selected Research

The science behind fish oil indicates that within three days it can penetrate plaque and make plaque less susceptible to rupture. Among the many studies, perhaps the most impressive is the ongoing GISSI trial in Italy. Researchers have followed more than eleven hundred Italians at 172 medical centers who experienced heart attacks. Included in the findings: individuals who took a 1 gram supplement of fish oil daily with a high concentration (850 mg of DHA/EPA) of omega-3 fatty acids had a 30 percent reduced risk of sudden cardiac death and all causes of death over a one-year period. This study was believed to influence the American Heart Association to recommend at least 1 gram of fish oil a day.

Our Recommendations

Use only pharmaceutical-grade fish oil supplements, which means purified products free of toxic substances such as mercury and PCBs (chlorinated compounds that contaminate the environment and accumulate in the bodies of fish and marine animals). Buy supplements from reputable manufacturers that ensure purity and that test their fish oil regularly for toxicity.

For prevention, take 1 gram a day. Patients with known CAD, stent, bypass, or a history of heart attack will benefit from higher dosages.

Some people prefer taking fish oil before bedtime because of the odor. You can take your fish oil once a day or throughout the day.

Generally speaking, these are well-tolerated supplements, although some people burp up the fish oil. If this is a problem, take the supplement with food or with digestive enzymes. Some fish oil supplements are specially coated, thereby eliminating the fish odor problem.

Precautions

Patients on Coumadin or other anticoagulants used to be told they should not take fish oil because it would make them bleed. While we advise prudent caution when combining fish oil or any other drug or nutritional agent with Coumadin, medical research indicates the two are compatible.

In one study, 610 patients who underwent successful coronary artery bypass surgery were randomized to receive Coumadin or aspirin, with or without 10 grams of fish oil per day. Supplementation did not increase the risk of abnormal bleeding, but interestingly it decreased the incidence of vein graft closure after one year by 25 percent—a superb benefit. Fish oil might actually decrease gastrointestinal tract bleeding risk. Research has shown that these fatty acids heal peptic ulcers nearly as well as prescription drugs.

If you take Coumadin and wish to take fish oil, discuss the situation with your doctor, who can monitor your clotting status and readjust your medication if necessary.

Having said that fish oil is not unsafe, there are certain situations in which you want to be a good clotter. For instance, if you have surgery coming up, stop the fish oil because of the potential for thinning the blood. Fish oil doesn't cause excess bleeding, but right after surgery you don't want it to slow down the clotting process. Resume fish oil after you heal, perhaps after three days. Always check with your doctor.

We recommend taking 2 mg daily of astaxanthin, an antioxidant with the ability to protect fish oils from oxidizing in your body. It has been our experience that fish oils can become oxidized in diabetics, whose bodies create considerable free radical stress. This effect can aggravate the condition. Taking fish oil along with an antioxidant helps keep blood sugar under control.

Magnesium

More than half of all Americans may be deficient in magnesium, a critical mineral. We find that most patients with CVD, especially acute disease, are depleted. Diabetics and postmenopausal women are extremely depleted.

Magnesium serves as a major partner in more than three hundred enzymatic reactions in the body, including the generation of cellular energy and muscle relaxation; the synthesis of fat, protein, and nucleic acids; and the maintenance of strong bones. Deficiency contributes to a wide range of symptoms, from muscle cramps and spasms, tics and tremors, and premenstrual difficulties to arrhythmias and sudden cardiac death.

It's hard for cardiologists not to be tuned in to magnesium because it helps so many of the routine conditions we treat: arterial disease, stroke, angina, heart attack, abnormal heart rhythms, cardiomyopathy and heart failure, high blood pressure, and mitral valve prolapse.

Magnesium is endothelial cell–friendly. Everybody with plaque should take it. It will stabilize plaque. Further research needs to be done to determine whether it reverses plaque.

Magnesium improves the metabolic efficiency of heart muscle cells, so it alleviates chest pain and other symptoms of angina due to lack of oxygen (ischemia). The mineral is particularly helpful in cases of ischemia caused by spasm of the coronary vessels because it helps relax the muscle walls of the arteries. It nurtures the heart during the acute phase of a heart attack, lowers soaring blood pressure that threatens to cause a stroke, and eases various cardiac arrhythmias that could develop into cardiac arrest.

Magnesium for Better Beating

Dr. Roberts: Among my patients with chronic CVD are individuals who experience uncomfortable arrhythmias—racing of the heart, or a condition of extra or skipped heartbeats that we call PVCs (premature ventricular complex). Every one of these patients has a magnesium deficiency. I give them all a magnesium supplement and their PVCs disappear. They all feel better. My staff personnel have become so aware of this effect that whenever a patient tests positive for PVCs they will let me know before I even see the patient that "so and so needs magnesium."

Why is magnesium deficiency so common? For one thing, the soil has become deficient in magnesium and other health-nurturing minerals. And then there's our lifestyle:

- Vegetables, nuts, and whole grains contain ample magnesium, but most people don't eat enough of them. The national preference for processed foods ensures a risky low magnesium intake. The refining of whole grains eliminates most of the magnesium content. For example, processing of whole wheat to white flour causes an 82 percent magnesium loss.

- High-fat diets generate soaps in the gut that wash out the magnesium in food.

- We take in too much calcium and too little magnesium, causing a mineral imbalance. Finland has the highest amount of calcium to magnesium in the diet—a 4 to 1 ratio—and the United States follows close behind. The Scandinavian country ranks first in the world in sudden death from heart attack and stroke among young to middle-aged men. Medical researchers believe a low magnesium intake has something to do with it.

- Alcohol, even in small amounts, drains magnesium. Alcoholics are woefully deficient.

- Colas and other soft drinks high in phosphates inactivate magnesium.

- Some parts of the United States, notably the Southeast, have low levels of magnesium in drinking water. Evidence suggests that magnesium-rich (hard) water may be the most bioavailable form of magnesium. Hard water areas have a lower heart attack rate than places where the water is soft.

- Stress depletes the body of magnesium. Any kind of stress has this effect: overwork, too much exercise or physical activity (athletes take note!), mental and emotional stress, surgery, or trauma (see chapter 11 for our discussion on stress and magnesium).

Selected Research

In 2003, researchers in Los Angeles, Austria, and Israel reported for the first time that magnesium supplementation significantly improved cardiac exercise tolerance and chest pain, as well as quality of life, in patients with CAD. The 187 patients in this study, already on medication programs, had been randomly assigned either a daily magnesium supplement (365 mg) or a placebo pill for six months.

The report, in the *American Journal of Cardiology*, attributed improvements to magnesium's multiple actions in the cardiovascular system, including protecting endothelial cells from calcium overload, promoting arterial dilation and relaxation, decreasing blood pressure, and enhancing ATP production in the mitochondria. Lead author Michael Shechter, of Israel's Sheba Medical Center Heart Institute, an international authority on magnesium therapy for CVD, noted that fully 75 percent of the patients with CAD he has studied in the United States and Israel have initial deficiencies of magnesium.

Shechter suggests that CAD itself may be related to magnesium deficiency. He believes that "this inexpensive and essentially safe nutritional supplement" should be part of all therapy programs for heart disease.

Shechter's findings help explain results in other important studies, such as the Honolulu Heart Program, in which researchers monitored the cardiovascular health over three decades of more than seven thousand men of Japanese ancestry living in Hawaii. Individuals with the lowest daily magnesium intake (50 to 186 mg) were almost twice as likely to have a heart attack than those with the highest average amount (340 to 1,183 mg). The RDA for men is around 400 mg and 300 mg for women.

Chronic magnesium deficiency probably plays an important role in the development of diabetes, a condition that carries with it many secondary health concerns, including an increased risk for CVD. In the large Women's Health Study, researchers tracked the health of 39,000 women forty-five and older for a six-year period. The women had no previous history of heart disease or diabetes. By the end of the study term, nearly 920 women had developed diabetes. The analysis of nutrient intake found a significant relationship between magnesium and diabetes. The higher the magnesium level, the lower the risk. Again, in two other major studies—involving 128,000 nurses and other health professionals—researchers found a similar magnesium intake connection. The exact mechanism by which magnesium lowers risk remains unclear, but we know that insulin resistance often improves with magnesium, and magnesium assists many diabetics to attain better glucose control.

Many people with insulin resistance have an accompanying risk factor of high triglycerides. Research indicates that the triglyceride level falls with increased magnesium, a direct effect we've observed in our patients many times. Magnesium, it turns out, directly feeds an important enzyme called lipoprotein lipase. The enzyme breaks down circulating triglycerides into fatty acids for tissue use and helps form beneficial HDL cholesterol.

Our Recommendations

To check for deficiency, ask your doctor for a red cell magnesium or ionized magnesium test. These tests yield more accurate measurements of functional magnesium. Standard blood-level magnesium tests often turn up falsely normal results.

If you take a diuretic, be alert that it causes excessive urinary loss of magnesium. Cardiovascular patients should take supplemental magnesium, especially diabetics, because it helps stabilize insulin levels, and as a result, helps stabilize plaque.

We recommend 400 to 800 mg a day, regardless of food intake. Some supplements come in tablet forms, others in chewable. We like the chewable form best because of superior absorbability.

Precautions

Too much magnesium acts as a laxative. You can often adjust your bowel movements just by how much magnesium you take. Quite frankly, this is a side effect that we count on with our elderly patients who complain of constipation. Bowel tolerance is an individual thing. If you are uncomfortable, reduce the dosage to get the cardiovascular benefits without the laxative effect.

Don't take extra magnesium if you suffer from kidney failure. The kidneys may not be able to excrete the mineral, which could contribute to a toxic buildup in the body.

Nattokinase and Lumbrokinase

Hyperviscosity refers to sticky or sludgy blood. When blood thickens, it bogs down as it moves through the blood vessels, causing platelets to stick together and clump. That puts strain on the heart to push blood through the system. Blood vessels become more rigid, less elastic, and frequently calcified. The danger lies in the tendency to form clots that can block vessels leading to the heart, brain, lungs, or other vital organs.

What causes thick blood?

- Genetics
- Aging
- Lack of exercise
- Too high a hematocrit level, a measure of red blood cell concentration. If hematocrit increases by 10 percent, viscosity can go up by 20 percent.
- Too much iron in the blood. Research shows that menstruating women have a lower incidence of heart disease, explained in part by losing blood and iron on a monthly basis. This correlates to lowered oxidative stress and blood viscosity. Men and older women who donate blood on a regular basis reduce the viscosity and risk for clogged vessels.
- Deformed red blood cells, a result of aging, diabetes, high homocysteine, and mechanical forces within vessels.
- Environmental toxins and cigarette smoke that pollute and inflame.

Obviously, you want optimum coagulability, less stagnation, and thus healthier arteries. We've already seen how one supplement—fish oil—helps keep blood thin. But many individuals, including those who choose to avoid pharmaceutical blood thinners, may need something even stronger. That's where nattokinase and lumbrokinase come in.

These enzymes are relatively new kids on the supplement block. As therapeutic agents, and even for prevention, they have us very excited.

Nattokinase is extracted from the traditional fermented soy food natto, believed by some researchers to contribute to the low incidence of coronary heart disease in Japan. Ralph E. Holsworth Jr., an osteopathic physician in Pagosa Springs, Colorado, introduced nattokinase in the United States. He suggests that nattokinase may significantly impact heart disease treatment because it "provides a unique, powerful, and safe way to eliminate clots, or reduce the tendency to form clots, and thus decrease the risk of heart attack and stroke."

Lumbrokinase, developed in both Japan and China, comes from an extract of earthworm, a traditional source of healing in Asian medicine.

These two separate products of dynamic Asian research share a powerful and common property of great interest to cardiologists: they wield a fibrin-degrading ability even stronger than the plasmin produced in the body. They are natural clot eaters.

Your body produces fibrin, a fibrous protein formed from fibrinogen. This main clotting factor creates a weblike mesh that snares red blood cells and thickens the blood so that you don't bleed excessively from an injury. Fibrin's clot-forming action becomes immediately activated when plaques rupture. It is part of the body's defense reaction to toxins suddenly pouring into the blood. So fibrin is both important and dangerous at the same time. Plaque ruptures aside, cardiologists become concerned whenever they see consistently thick blood as a result of excess fibrin activity.

To offset the danger and create blood viscosity balance, the body naturally produces plasmin, an enzyme that breaks down excess fibrin. If this natural anticlotting agent becomes overwhelmed and can't do the job, there is trouble. And that's where nattokinase and lumbrokinase come in.

Holsworth has personally used nattokinase supplements in more than five hundred cases. "For me, it has been of significant therapeutic value in treating high blood pressure, ischemic stroke, and peripheral artery disease, and dissolving deep vein thrombosis," he says. "Administered soon after severe strokes, it may help restore some of the lost functions. I've been able to help many diabetic patients with eye and kidney problems, as well as postpone the need for amputations."

Moreover, Holsworth reports, nattokinase works effectively as a natural option for patients who cannot use Coumadin or heparin, and preventively for people with thrombophilia, a largely genetic predisposition to form clots. Abnormal clot formation contributes significantly to deaths in the United States—more than six hundred thousand Americans each year. An estimated 5 to 7 percent of Caucasians of European descent in the United States have an increased tendency for thrombosis.

Clots comprise much of the content of plaque. So if we can dissolve the clotted material, we can open arteries and improve blood flow. If you reduce the clot just a tiny bit, you get a significant boost to blood flow. You might even say you are removing the vulnerability from plaque. Nattokinase and lumbrokinase are oral clot busters, and they work within minutes to hours. If you take these supplements preventively, you may not form clots in the first place.

Clot Busters at Work

Dr. Roberts has been using lumbrokinase and find it generates the same effect as nattokinase, eating away at clots and preventing the consequences of plaque rupture. He recalls one of his elderly male patients who was diagnosed with CAD and came to see him about an increase in chest pain, a case of unstable angina. The patient was on a medication program, but the threat still existed of plaque rupture and an acute event. Here was a potential time bomb ready to explode.

The patient refused to be hospitalized for an angiogram, so Dr. Roberts put him on lumbrokinase. The chest pain quickly eased, apparently because the supplement digested the clot. The acute pain didn't return.

Another patient, a woman, was rushed to Dr. Roberts's office by her husband. She was having a TIA—a mini-stroke. Her speech was slurred, her face numb, and her hand movements awkward. She refused hospitalization. Dr. Roberts immediately gave her a couple of lumbrokinase capsules with a sip of water and then examined her. In a few moments, her speech normalized. She was soon able to leave the office without assistance. With a prescription for lumbrokinase and the antiplatelet medication Plavix, she rapidly stabilized.

She was not, however, the most compliant patient. Several times, she discontinued the supplement and her symptoms returned. She had a serious clotting problem that the lumbrokinase helped keep in check. Eventually she got the message.

Selected Research

Two large multihospital studies from China have demonstrated improvement from lumbrokinase in unstable angina and return of function following stroke. The research indicates a reduction in blood viscosity and, in the case of stroke, heightened recovery from nervous system damage if taken within a month of the event. Lumbrokinase has been used in Chinese hospitals since the early 1990s.

Nattokinase has been the subject of seventeen studies, including two small human trials. In one, volunteers who received 200 grams of nattokinase before breakfast showed a heightened ability to dissolve blood clots. On average, the volunteers' ELT (euglobulin lysis time, a measure of how long it takes to dissolve a blood clot) dropped by 48 percent within two hours of treatment, and volunteers retained an enhanced ability to dissolve blood clots for two to eight hours.

In another study, Italian researchers used a nattokinase supplement to reduce thrombotic events such as deep vein thrombosis among high-risk individuals with thrombophilia during and after prolonged airline flights. Blood coagulability increases during long air travel and blood flow slows down, especially in the lower legs. Dehydration and in-flight alcohol exacerbate the situation.

Our Recommendations

Nattokinase and lumbrokinase have a great future in both preventing and treating atherosclerotic buildup. Since our natural production of plasmin slows as we age and other factors can enter the picture to thicken the blood, it makes good sense to consider these enzymes for prevention.

We strongly recommend them for people at high risk for forming clots. If you have high fibrinogen, homocysteine, Lp(a), and CRP levels, you may want to seriously consider this option with your doctor. One of the most lethal combinations we see in our practices is elevated homocysteine and Lp(a). These toxic blood overloads put patients at high risk to make excess fibrin.

If you take medication, ask your physician before starting either of these enzyme supplements. They are quite powerful and your medication may have to be adjusted as a result of taking them.

Lumbrokinase is marketed by Canada RNA (www.canadarna.com) and sold through the company's Web site. You can readily find nattokinase in health food stores.

We suggest the following dosages:

- Nattokinase: For prevention, 2,000 fibrin units per day. For therapy, 4,000 units per day. Following a stroke, 6,000 units.

- Lumbrokinase: Active therapy involves two 20 mg capsules taken thirty minutes before meals, three times a day for four weeks. Then one capsule three times a day. If taken with food, lumbrokinase will serve as a digestive enzyme and none will be absorbed into the blood. Those with high fibrinogen and Lp(a) levels should take one capsule at bedtime.

Precautions

If you take Coumadin, don't take either of these supplements without approval from your doctor. They can be used with aspirin and Plavix (an anticlotting medication), but with caution and under a doctor's supervision. Stop taking nattokinase and lumbrokinase two days prior to surgery and don't resume until about two weeks afterward.

L-arginine

The most important determinant of cardiovascular well-being—or lack of it—is the biochemical health of the endothelium, the single layer of cells lining the interior wall of the blood vessels. You'll likely be fine if you have a significant narrowing of your coronary arteries but good endothelial function. If you have a 40 percent narrowing but terrible endothelial function, your prospects are poor. Biochemistry supercedes anatomy. It determines cardiovascular life or death.

By biochemistry, we mean the ability of these cells to function as hormone factories, particularly to produce nitric oxide, a compound that relaxes the arteries, keeps them flexible, and promotes blood flow. Nitroglycerin, the traditional medication to relieve chest pains, is simply a drug form of nitric oxide.

As we age, we make less nitric oxide. Deficiency permits blood vessels to constrict and lose their flexibility, contributing to vessel stiffness, inflammation and plaque buildup, and hypertension. Moreover, a vicious cycle develops: increased blood pressure and inflammation impair the ability of the endothelial cells to make nitric oxide.

Above and beyond these central effects, nitric oxide's biggest claim to

fame is its connection to Viagra, the popular drug used for erectile dysfunction (ED). Viagra promotes the action of nitric oxide to help relax
blood vessels and vascular smooth muscle tissue in the penis. The result:
increased blood flow and a harder erection. It is interesting to note that
Viagra was developed originally for CVD. It didn't work for that purpose
because it increases the nitric oxide effect only in the penis and the eyes,
and possibly in the pulmonary artery in kids with congenital heart disease.
Some research has indicated that men with ED as a result of reduced
nitric oxide may be at increased risk for CVD.

To make nitric oxide, the body needs L-arginine, an amino acid found
in many foods such as dairy products, meat, poultry, fish, nuts, seeds, and
chocolate. If you take in a lot of L-arginine, you make more nitric oxide
and obtain greater protection against the damaging effects of diabetes,
smoking, high blood pressure, free radical stress, and many of the problems related to CVD.

L-arginine: The "Poor/Smart Man's Viagra"

Dr. Sinatra: L-arginine is like the "poor man's Viagra" in a way. Before I knew
about the arterial dilation connection between nitric oxide and L-arginine, I
used to recommend 8 grams of L-arginine to patients to help lower cholesterol. Then I started getting excited feedback from my male patients that they
would wake up with firm erections in the morning. That can happen at high
dosage. At lower dosages, we don't get the potency boost, but we do get
endothelial improvement.

Selected Research

L-arginine was first found to boost nitric oxide and arterial physiology in
a series of Stanford studies published in 1992. Rabbits with high cholesterol levels supplemented with L-arginine developed significant improvement in arterial and endothelial function compared to nonsupplemented
animals. L-arginine appeared to help defuse the biochemical events that
initiate atherosclerosis.

Later, in another rabbit study, German researchers showed that
L-arginine supplementation started after the formation of plaque not
only improved arterial dilation but also stopped plaque progression.
Moreover, they found that L-arginine had a much greater effect than

Mevacor, a popular statin drug, which actually increased endothelial free radical activity.

Other studies have shown that L-arginine:

- Reduces endothelial dysfunction irrespective of the cause

- Provides an antioxidant effect

- Blocks LDL oxidation

- Blocks platelet clumping and white cell adhesion to the vascular wall

- Decreases angina frequency and nitroglycerin need

- Improves symptoms in patients with heart failure

- Improves outcome following heart attack

- Improves functional status in patients with coronary and/or lower extremity vascular blockages

Our Recommendations

L-arginine has value for the whole gamut of atherosclerosis—from early signs such as high blood pressure and erectile dysfunction to advanced cardiac events. We feel it offers promise for plaque stabilization and reversal. It is inexpensive and nontoxic. We both use it clinically for treating angina, high blood pressure, erectile dysfunction, and stubborn risk factors we can't otherwise improve.

Suggested dosage: 2,000 to 3,000 mg three times daily. To affect penis potency, take a single 8 gram dose at bedtime.

L-arginine can be purchased as capsules or tablets in health food stores. You may want to obtain it as a bulk powder and mix it in juice, smoothies, or warm water. Be aware that the taste is not pleasant. See the supplement section in appendix A for more information.

Precautions

In a 2006 issue of the *Journal of the American Medical Association*, Johns Hopkins researchers reported on the use of L-arginine during the six months following a heart attack. They compared the results of daily supplementation versus placebo on 153 patients to determine whether L-arginine decreased arterial stiffness and improved ejection fraction, the measure of how much blood the left ventricle of the heart pumps out with each contraction.

The published results were negative—to our surprise. The researchers used 9 grams daily of L-arginine with standard medication. They found no improvement in arterial stiffness or ejection fraction and reported six deaths among older patients (over 60 years of age) randomized to take the supplements, prompting an early termination of the study. No such deaths occurred in the placebo group. They concluded that "L-arginine therapy should not be given to patients following a myocardial infarction."

This was the first negative article on L-arginine we have encountered in the medical literature. L-arginine is part of our routine recommendation for patients because of its desirable nitric oxide effect that we discussed earlier. It's an endothelial-friendly nutrient. The researchers did not find this effect, however, in their post–heart attack patients.

In our practices, we do not prescribe L-arginine right after a heart attack. We emphasize L-carnitine, CoQ10, magnesium, and fish oil—supplements documented by research to be extremely beneficial and safe during and after heart attacks and that enhance outcomes and survivability substantially.

Cardiologists are aware of a particular vulnerability in patients six months to a year after a heart attack. We wonder if the L-arginine used by itself during the time frame in this study may have created a problem among the participants that was previously not known, and thus as a single supplement proved to be ineffective and somehow detrimental in a severely diseased arterial environment.

We never recommend L-arginine or any other supplement alone. Our patients take foundational supplements containing a broad range of vitamins, minerals, and antioxidants, plus targeted nutrients for specific healing effects. Could a high dose of L-arginine by itself in this experiment could have generated excess free radicals that might have had a damaging effect that was not neutralized by taking antioxidants? There could also be an unknown confounding effect associated with heavy post–heart attack medication.

It is also interesting to note that in the Johns Hopkins study, the cause of death of two of the six patients was sepsis (infection), something apparently unrelated to L-arginine. This outcome edges the mortality incidence toward the direction of borderline, a "possible" increased risk in older patients, the researchers said, adding that the results might also have been due to chance.

It is unfortunate that the authors never acknowledged other studies on L-arginine that have been highly positive and shown benefits for post–heart attack, unstable angina, and heart failure patients.

Whether this study is correct or flawed, we don't know. But it has been published and a red flag raised regarding the use of L-arginine alone right after heart attacks. Until we hear otherwise, we will not recommend L-arginine as part of a general supplementation program for about six months or so after a cardiac event. Any patient who wants to resume this supplement after a heart attack should do so only under the supervision of a cardiologist.

Don't use L-arginine if you have a herpes infection. It might also stimulate an outbreak, in which case you could take lysine, an antagonistic amino acid. L-arginine might also make migraines worse because of the arterial dilation effect.

Phosphatidylcholine (Essential Phospholipids)

Cellular membranes function as the interface between the machinery inside of cells and the extracellular fluid that bathes all cells. If all is well, the two-way traffic through the membranes involves nutrients entering to sustain the activities inside while waste products exit.

Fats (lipids) and proteins make up the cell membranes. If the fatty acids in your diet are predominantly unsaturated fat (from vegetables and fish oil), cell membranes maintain a desirable elasticity and permeability. Traffic flows in and out. However, if you eat too much saturated fat (as in meat and dairy) or trans fats (hydrogenated and fried oils), your membranes stiffen up and the cell has trouble exchanging nutrients for wastes.

Membrane lipids include cholesterol and a fatty substance called phosphatidylcholine (two fatty acids bound to the molecules of phosphorus and choline). We'll refer to it as PC. The health of the membrane also depends on the ratio of PC to cholesterol. Red blood cells with too much cholesterol and not enough PC become rigid and have trouble moving through the capillaries of our microcirculation.

Platelets with a low PC-to-cholesterol ratio are more likely to form inappropriate blood clots. Red cell and platelet membranes rich in PC, however, function as nature intended. PC is a vital raw material for the transmission of nerve impulses and processing of cholesterol.

Although your body makes choline, a primary constituent of PC, you still have to consume some in your diet to maintain health. The most common source of choline is lecithin, a special kind of fat called a phospholipid that is found in egg yolks, liver, peanuts, wheat germ, cauliflower, milk, and soybeans. As a heart-healthy nutritional supplement, lecithin was wildly popular about twenty-five years ago.

Lecithin promotes reverse cholesterol transport, the process by which HDL escorts LDL cholesterol out of the arterial wall and back to the liver for elimination. Lecithin serves as a needed raw material for HDL.

Years ago, a German pharmaceutical firm developed a method to extract a specific PC from soy lecithin. The extract was used in Europe in the treatment of liver disease, high cholesterol, CVD, and certain neurological impairments. This preparation, referred to as essential phospholipid (EPL), produces a significantly greater therapeutic effect than straight lecithin.

Selected Research

Essential phospholipid has been used for more than two decades in Europe to improve cell membrane function and the cholesterol profile. It also improves insulin resistance, lowers blood viscosity, and has an anticlotting activity. It keeps platelets from sticking.

In animal experiments, EPL has generated actual reversal of atherosclerotic plaque. In humans, a lessening of CVD manifestations was documented with long-term treatment: less angina and less claudication. Provisional clinical results suggest a possible decrease in the size of atherosclerotic plaque. More than a thousand articles and abstracts have been published documenting EPL's efficacy.

Our Recommendations

Essential phospholipid for intravenous use is available from European pharmacies under the trade names of Lipostabil and Essentiale and from compounding pharmacies in the United States. Treatment effects are phenomenal, but the cost of treatment is quite high. An average patient requires twenty to forty treatments at about $150 per IV treatment.

The good news: oral EPL supplements are available. The one that absorbs the best is DetoxMaxPlus, sold to doctors through BioImmune in Scottsdale, Arizona (888-663-8844). BioImmune will not sell the product directly to the public. It is too strong to be used without a doctor's supervision. The company can provide interested patients with the name of a doctor familiar with the product.

DetoxMaxPlus contains PC in combination with EDTA, a synthetic amino acid that binds toxic metals and helps remove them from the body (see chapter 8 for more information). A high-speed agitation process renders the PC particles so small that they readily absorb through the gut and into the cells, where they then release the embedded EDTA.

The combination of ingredients, along with enhanced absorption, yields impressive therapeutic benefit. Along with PC, you get heavy metal removal, and thus help neutralize another source of inflammation and plaque.

We recommend DetoxMaxPlus to patients with symptomatic CVD, certainly for anyone with plaque and resistant cases of inoperable heart disease where nothing else has worked well. We see general improvement, including better blood flow and a reduced heavy metal load. Keep in mind that we use this supplement with the rest of our program, not as a solo therapy.

As a trial, six of our patients with longstanding CVD underwent carotid artery ultrasound testing before and after taking DetoxMaxPlus and lumbrokinase for twenty weeks. Blood flow improved. Some of our patients experienced improvement in angina as well.

DetoxMaxPlus comes in two-ounce bottles. Take a half ounce twice a week on an empty stomach for twenty to forty weeks. Then cut back to a half ounce every two weeks, the long-term maintenance dosage. The cost: $50 per two-ounce bottle.

Precautions

Your physician needs to monitor kidney function while you take an oral chelator. That's because it removes toxic metals, including mercury, which can be stressful to the kidneys. We don't recommend oral chelators for individuals with serious kidney dysfunction or for pregnant women.

Vitamin C

Most people taking vitamin C for protection from colds would never guess that they are getting a big heart and artery boost to boot. Consider these benefits of vitamin C:

- Retards progression of atherosclerosis. For people with this disease, it decreases the incidence of adverse cardiovascular events and related deaths by 40 to 60 percent.

- Decreases the need for repeat angioplasty by 57 percent.

- Reverses endothelial dysfunction.

- Improves recovery after bypass surgery and cuts the risk of post-operative atrial fibrillation in half.

- Improves recovery following heart attack.

- Helps control blood pressure.

- Keeps CRP in check.

- Helps neutralize Lp(a) and vascular wall damage due to homocysteine.

- Promotes conversion of excess cholesterol into bile acids that aid in the digestion of fats.

- Gets the lead out of your system.

Do you know of any other medication that can do so much?

Mammals—with the exception of bats, guinea pigs, and, most notably, human beings—make vitamin C in the liver. Humans must obtain it through diet—from foods such as fruits and vegetables—or through supplementation. Vitamin C deficiency leads to weakness, poor immunity, internal hemorrhage, and an unraveling of the connective tissue that binds the nuts and bolts of the body. Outright deficiency is called scurvy. Less than a full-blown deficiency but enough of a deficit to shortchange the body is referred to as subclinical scurvy, a widespread chronic condition that the two-time Nobel Prize laureate Linus Pauling considered the underlying cause of CVD. We can become depleted from smoking, poor diet, medications, aging, and stress.

The body needs vitamin C to make collagen, the primary structural protein of the connective tissue holding together your entire physical structure. It thus has a hand in making arteries more elastic and tougher so that they can better resist mechanical forces and inflammatory insult.

Vitamin C improves dilation of atherosclerotic blood vessels, a benefit for individuals with angina, heart failure, high cholesterol, and high blood pressure. Improved blood flow has been documented in studies at a daily dosage of 500 mg.

Vitamin C is also a potent antioxidant and offers protection to proteins, lipids, carbohydrates, and even DNA from damage by free radicals. It protects endothelial cells from the oxidative damage of homocysteine and also boosts the activity of glutathione, the powerful antioxidant produced in the body.

We have talked about Lp(a) in detail before. This troublesome cholesterol particle is highly inflammatory and thrombotic, and it is a difficult risk factor to overcome. Vitamin C helps us neutralize it. Fish oil, L-carnitine, L-lysine, and proline help here as well.

For CVD patients, vitamin C is a must-have supplement. And, as the evolution of medical research indicates, it can help keep you out of cardiovascular trouble to begin with.

Selected Research

In 1940, the Ottawa pathologist J. C. Patterson demonstrated that heart attacks were not primarily due to atherosclerotic plaque buildup within the wall of the coronary arteries but rather to destabilization or rupture of the fibrous cap covering the plaque. A year later, he suggested the cause of such destabilization was vitamin C deficiency.

During World War II, the Nobel Prize laureate Sir Hans Krebs in England found he could create chest pain and EKG evidence of coronary distress when previously healthy young people were fed diets exceptionally low in vitamin C.

Then, in the early 1950s, G. C. Willis, another Canadian pathologist, discovered abnormal vitamin C content in the arteries of individuals who died of CVD. In a series of follow-up experiments, Willis placed guinea pigs on a low vitamin C diet. Guinea pigs, like humans, cannot make vitamin C. The animals all developed arterial disease, which subsequently reversed when Willis added vitamin C back to their chow. He postulated that vitamin C deficiency was a critical factor in atherosclerosis.

In his pathology research, Willis observed at autopsy that all patients with advanced coronary disease and prior heart attack also had evidence of atherosclerotic plaque buildup in their femoral and popliteal arteries (the arteries to the legs, between the groin and the back of the knee). He felt that arterial changes in this area of the body, which he could visualize with angiography, reflected similar changes in the coronary arteries. At that point in time, coronary artery angiography was unavailable in Montreal, where Willis worked. The pathologist was convinced that vitamin C deficiency played a major role in the atherosclerosis process and that supplementation could modify the course of disease. To test his hypothesis, he and his associates at Montreal General Hospital carried out femoral-popliteal angiographic studies in twenty-two middle-aged men with symptomatic CVD or diabetes. Using 500 mg of vitamin C three times a day over a period of up to six months, the researchers actually decreased the arterial plaque and symptoms in some of the individuals—an extraordinary accomplishment by 1954 standards.

Willis's research showed that vitamin C alone could significantly improve patients with advanced disease. He concluded that vitamin C is "essential for the maintenance of the ground substance [connective tissue] of the arterial intima. Any factor disturbing [its] metabolism either systemically or locally results in ground substance injury with subsequent lipid deposit. The disturbance is of major importance in the pathogenesis of arterial calcification, intimal hemorrhaging, and thrombosis." The antidote was simple, he said: vitamin C.

Although forgotten today by most of the medical community, Patterson and Willis had made great discoveries. Vitamin C worked back then . . . and still works. A recent study in Italy confirmed the magnificent healing powers of vitamin C for arterial disease. In the study, researchers monitored a thousand individuals for more than ten years who had varying degrees of atherosclerotic plaque of the carotid and lower extremity arteries. The group was randomly divided in half at the outset: half took 1,000 mg daily of vitamin C; the other half took no supplement. Periodic ultrasounds were done.

The results, published in 2002, revealed that 13 percent of the non-supplemented individuals with minor plaque at the beginning experienced progression to visible plaque during the decade; in the vitamin C group, only 3 percent. For moderate initial plaque, such as a 20 percent narrowing, the incidence of deterioration was 38 percent without vitamin C and 8 percent with it. Among subjects with a greater than 50 percent baseline narrowing, two-thirds of the nonsupplemented group deteriorated as compared to only 21 percent of those who took vitamin C.

The study dramatically showed a major delay in progression and a blunting of the disease process over ten years from vitamin C alone. Moreover, the mortality rate was 43 percent less in the vitamin group!

Vitamin C, and for that matter all of the nutritional and pharmacologic agents that we use to benefit the heart patient, do not work primarily by opening up the artery but rather by protecting the narrowed artery from plaque rupture, spasm, and clot formation. They favorably affect blood flow rate and the functional integrity of the endothelial cells lining the artery.

We recommend the whole range of antioxidants to our patients. Nevertheless, the studies showing the singular effects of supplements like vitamin C are extremely impressive.

Our Recommendations

Most every adult should take 1,000 mg of vitamin C as part of a daily supplement regimen. We often recommend larger doses for patients, depending on their Lp(a) and CRP levels, and our estimate of their degree of arterial inflammation. For best results, split the dosages into two or three servings throughout the day. If you are forgetful, it is better to take 1,000 mg in one dose rather than to forget subsequent dosages.

Some skeptics maintain that more than 200 mg per day is worthless. It just creates "expensive urine," they say. But a recent analysis of nine major studies shows that people who take more than 700 mg per day have about 30 percent less CVD mortality compared to nonvitamin users. Consumers can hardly find a pill today providing less than 500 mg of vitamin C. While true that much of the vitamin passes out in the urine soon after you take it orally, much of it enters your cells. Probably what does go out has performed an antioxidant or detoxifying function traveling through your body.

Vitamin C enhances iron absorption and thus may be of additional value to menstruating women, but in men and postmenopausal women this effect represents some concern. You need enough iron in your diet to make a normal complement of red blood cells, but beyond that iron has negative health effects. Free iron, not participating in hemoglobin formation or other iron-requiring biochemical processes, acts as a free radical, promoting the oxidation of LDL and other intracellular and extracellular structures. Iron excess is associated with endothelial dysfunction, insulin resistance, and an increased risk for cardiovascular disease. To be on the safe side, check for evidence of iron overload with a serum ferritin lab test.

What type of vitamin C should you take? Vitamin C's chemical name is ascorbic acid, and yes, if you have a sensitive stomach, it might cause some irritation. If plain ascorbic acid bothers you, consider a buffered or mineral ascorbate form that tends to be gentler on the stomach. One such version is sodium ascorbate, used and recommended for many years by Linus Pauling.

Bioflavonoids (also known as vitamin P) help escort vitamin C into the body. These compounds, found in fruits and vegetables, have beneficial effects of their own. It's worth it to pay a little more for a vitamin C supplement complexed with bioflavonoids. Esterified vitamin C (Ester C) is better absorbed than regular vitamin C, but it costs more.

The bottom line: it doesn't really matter which vitamin C you take. Just take it. Find a preparation you tolerate well and can easily afford.

Vitamin C represents a very inexpensive way to reduce Lp(a). For people with a high Lp(a) level and known coronary disease, we recommend 1,000 mg for every 10 points of Lp(a). So if you test at 50 mg/dl, for instance, we would suggest 5,000 mg of vitamin C. We like to see a level below 30, ideally below 20. Vitamin C may not always bring down the Lp(a) value, but patients do well on it. For patients experiencing repeated problems, we also recommend 500 to 1,000 mg each of the amino acids proline and L-lysine. This is purely observational on our part, but we see improvement from these additional supplements.

If you take vitamin C the night before open heart surgery, the risk of developing postoperative atrial fibrillation drops by more than half—from 33 percent to 14 percent—compared to someone who doesn't supplement. This conclusion is based on a Cleveland Clinic study in which individuals took 2,000 mg the night before surgery and then 500 mg twice a day during their postoperative recovery.

Cigarette smoke destroys vitamin C in the body, one of the means by which smoking promotes cardiovascular disease. Smokers thus have a greater need for vitamin C and consequently a more robust treatment benefit.

Attention, Nitroglycerin Users

Unhealthy endothelial cells don't make enough nitric oxide. That's why angina patients have been using nitroglycerin tablets for more than fifty years. The tablet delivers a dollop of nitric oxide to the arteries to keep the blood vessels dilated and prevent spasm and the clumping of platelets.

In recent times, cardiologists have prescribed nitroglycerin in sustained-release and patch forms to provide a constant supply of nitric oxide and prevent additional attacks of angina throughout the day. Patients have not needed to take as many under-the-tongue tablets.

However, convenience comes at a price. These long-lasting preparations aggravate underlying endothelial dysfunction by disturbing a key enzyme system. Here's the scenario: Endothelial cells produce nitric oxide synthase, an enzyme that converts L-arginine into nitric oxide. Whenever a person takes nitroglycerin, his or her nitric oxide level shoots up. Idleness is the devil's playground, they say, and so now the suddenly unneeded and out-of-work enzyme creates mischief by converting oxygen into a nasty free radical called superoxide. Superoxide neutralizes nitric oxide, whether from the medication or from endothelial cells, promoting blood vessel constriction and platelet stickiness.

In health, your body routinely performs countless balancing acts among countless enzymatic reactions. The give-and-take between nitric oxide and superoxide is one example. Another scenario for CVD occurs when this particular balancing act goes awry. The short-acting nitroglycerin tab provides symptom relief, an upside, but the continual action of the long-acting nitroglycerin upsets the balance: the patient gets an upside plus a nullifying superoxide downside. Symptoms recur. The doctor increases the dosage of the long-acting nitroglycerin. This helps for a while, but the endothelial cells now produce more damaging superoxide and little or no nitric oxide on their own. The nitric oxide is degraded. Symptoms return.

We call this nitrate tolerance, but in reality we are dealing with drug-induced endothelial dysfunction. The intent was good. We relieve symptoms but in the process damage the endothelium, actually increasing the risk for future adverse events.

Vitamin C along with vitamin E and N-acetylcysteine (another antioxidant nutritional supplement with lung and kidney protective benefits) prevent nitrate tolerance. When taken together, you get the upside without the downside. We recommend 1,000 mg of vitamin C with 500 mg of N-acetylcysteine or 200 to 400 IU of vitamin E.

B Vitamins

The Miracle of Niacin

Prior to his heart attack, Lou epitomized destructive type A behavior. He was a young, ambitious salesman for a major company. He traveled a lot, pushed himself, was under a lot of stress, worked long hours, and made a lot of money. He didn't know how to relax.

At a routine physical checkup, his doctor picked up on a somewhat high cholesterol level (257) and a low HDL count. Lou was advised to follow a low-fat diet and he duly minimized his fat intake. In doing so, however, he fell into the common pitfall of a replacement diet loaded with processed foods high in trans-fatty acids and sugar.

After the switch, Lou's cholesterol decreased to about 210. Nothing wrong with that. But his HDL level also dropped, from 33 to 29—the lowest in his life. We like to see men no lower than 35, and women no lower than 40. Low HDL is a serious risk factor for heart problems. It is the component of cholesterol that picks up harmful oxidized LDL and transports it back to the liver for removal.

Lou's new diet was really a time bomb for disaster. Trans fats lower HDL and stoke free radical damage to cell membranes, injury that kindles inflammation, disease, and age-related changes. They also promote LDL oxidation and raise Lp(a).

Lou was extremely vulnerable because of his low HDL level, which became even lower on a poorly designed diet. Six months later he had a heart attack. It was his wake-up call.

Lou looked for a preventive cardiologist and started consulting with Dr. Sinatra. Today, seven years later, he looks great at age forty-two, the result of a lifestyle program designed to put him back on the health track. He still has the same demanding sales job but has infused more balance into his life. He makes time to exercise and play with his kids. He avoids sugar and processed foods while eating plenty of good protein and healthy fats from olive oil, walnuts, and almonds.

Plus he takes niacin (vitamin B-3), a fabulous supplement for raising HDL. When Dr. Sinatra first saw Lou, his HDL level was 31. At a recent checkup it was 68.

Niacin has been a pillar of our supplement program for years. Lars Carlson of the Karolinska Institute in Stockholm calls niacin a "miracle drug" for all the lipid disorders that are risk factors for atherosclerosis.

Niacin lowers the levels of LDL cholesterol and Lp(a), and, as Dr. Carlson points out, "it raises more than any other drug the levels of the protective HDL lipoproteins."

Many studies have shown that treatment with niacin reduces progression of atherosclerosis and clinical events and mortality associated with coronary heart disease.

We prescribe the traditional form of niacin—the kind that causes the pins-and-needles flushing sensation. Some people feel discomforted by the flushing, but if you can tolerate it, and most people do, this is the way to raise HDL. It's the only one we know of that does it consistently well.

Our Recommendations

Lou takes 3 grams a day of niacin. That's a lot, but he needed it to get his HDL back on track. We usually find that 1½ to 2 grams is enough for most people to raise low HDL into a healthy zone. No medical drug can

All about the Niacin Flush

A tingly, pins-and-needles, sometimes hot, flushing of the skin primarily on the face, arms, and chest is common when you take niacin. It can occur initially at doses as low as 50 mg a day.

The flush begins in the forehead and works its way down the body. The higher the initial dose the greater is the initial flush. The intensity of the flush is minimized by taking the pills after meals.

Niacin causes small blood vessels—called capillaries—to increase in size. When this happens near the surface of the skin, the area turns reddish and feels hot and tingly. The flush usually lasts no more than a half-hour to an hour, and then disappears.

We have had patients over the years who became so alarmed that they went to the emergency room. You will think you are having some kind of a bad physical reaction. However, it is nothing to be concerned about.

We asked Abram Hoffer about the flush. Hoffer, a retired psychiatrist in Victoria, British Columbia, codiscovered niacin's cholesterol-lowering properties more than fifty years ago and subsequently used it for thousands of patients over decades. He found it also greatly benefits schizophrenics.

Hoffer said the flush is most intense initially. As you continue taking niacin, the intensity lessens, and often within a week or two it vanishes completely. If you stop taking niacin and then resume at some later date you may experience a full flush again.

"I have been taking niacin for fifty-five years, and except for the first few times I never flushed again," he said. "But everyone is individual, and the intensity and frequency can be affected by different factors. Anyone taking niacin for the first time should be aware that flushing may occur."

Some people use the nonflush form of niacin because they are uncomfortable with the flushing effect. The problem with that is you don't get the same good vascular benefits. There are different kinds of nonflush niacin. They tend to be expensive. If you want reliable results though, you should use the standard niacin, which is very inexpensive, according to Dr. Hoffer.

---

do that now, although we envision a time in the near future when we will have medication specifically for that.

You may want to start at a lower dosage, such as 250 mg three times a day after meals. Then work your way up gradually to a higher dosage.

Precautions

Niacin is very safe; however, many people have been reluctant to take it because of a supposed liver problem. We have never encountered that in practice and so we asked niacin expert Abram Hoffer his opinion. His answer:

"Among the many myths perpetuated about the dangers of vitamins is that niacin causes liver disease. Unfortunately, many physicians are afraid to use a high dose of niacin because of this unfounded fear. To me this is a tragedy because of all the patients who could be benefiting and who are not. A real liver connection just doesn't exist. There have been a few rare cases reported, the last serious one perhaps thirty or forty years ago.

"I have never encountered a liver problem using high-dose niacin for more than a half century. If I thought for a minute it could cause liver disease, I wouldn't take it. One of my patients is 112 years old, the second oldest person in Canada. She was doing cross-country skiing until two years ago. She has been taking niacin for forty-two years. Another patient asked me once what was the major danger from taking this vitamin. I answered that you'll live longer."

Hoffer says that in some patients niacin increases the values in liver function tests. It is assumed, incorrectly, that such results means underlying liver problems. If you are scheduled to take a liver function test, you may want to stop taking niacin five days beforehand in order to avoid possible confusion.

B Vitamins and Homocysteine

More than three decades ago, the New England pathologist Kilmer McCully postulated that homocysteine triggers arterial disease by instigating plaque and blood clot formation. His courageous persistence, in contradiction to the reigning cholesterol theory, got him booted out of two university jobs, and he was dismissed by the medical establishment for years. Gradually, however, McCully's theory was validated by researchers throughout the world. Today, elevated homocysteine is widely recognized as a major risk factor for CVD.

The homocysteine problem stems from a deficiency of three B-complex vitamins—B-6, folic acid, and B-12—that prevent proper processing of dietary protein. B-6 and folic acid have been typically deficient in the standard American diet filled with nutrient-poor processed foods. On any given day, more than 50 percent of adults fail to eat the recommended three servings of vegetables, and only 24 percent eat the recommended two servings of fruit. Fruits and vegetables are excellent sources of vitamins B-6 and folic acid.

In 1998, the U.S. Food and Drug Administration mandated supplementation of folic acid to grains, cereals, rice, pasta, and bread in an effort to curb the incidence of neural tube defects, a deficiency-related condition causing malformation of the spine or the head in newborns. Nevertheless, folic acid and B-6 deficiencies are still common. So, too, is B-12 deficiency, particularly in the elderly due to a decline in the production of stomach acid.

Selected Research

McCully's homocysteine theory received a breakthrough boost in the early 1990s from evidence emerging out of the famous Framingham Heart Study. Researchers found that older individuals deficient in folic acid, B-6, and B-12 had a higher homocysteine level. The research also showed a connection with narrowing of the carotid arteries. Homocysteine tends to rise slowly with aging. Later in the 1990s, and among a younger population, published data from the Nurses' Health Study conducted by the Harvard School of Public Health revealed that the lower the intake of folic acid and B-6, the greater the risk of death from CVD.

Continuing research has shown that supplementation, most effectively with folic acid, rapidly normalizes homocysteine levels in the blood, resulting in improved endothelial function. A 2002 study from Switzerland, reported in the *Journal of the American Medical Association*, described significant benefits for patients after coronary angioplasty to open arteries in and around the heart. Two hundred and five patients were divided randomly to receive either a daily placebo or a combination of 1 mg of folic acid, 10 mg of B-6, and 400 mcg of vitamin B-12. After six months, the vitamins were discontinued and a follow-up angiogram was carried out.

The researchers found 38 percent of the placebo-treated patients had renarrowed, compared to only 19 percent of the patients on B vitamins. Restenosis was reduced by 50 percent, as was the need for repeat angioplasty. No drug can do this! Cardiologists recognize the first three to six months as the riskiest for underlying plaque in a stretched vessel to reblock the artery. Plaque and fatty tissue tend to rebuild in the same arterial areas where angioplasty is performed, so the procedure may need to be repeated in the future. By lowering homocysteine and improving endothelial function, the B vitamins provide remarkable protection. At one year, these benefits were maintained. Moreover, the supplemented patients had a 15 percent complication rate (heart attack, bypass surgery, or death) during the year compared to 23 percent for the nonsupplemented patients.

In another 2002 study, researchers at King's College in London set out to see if folic acid alone could reduce homocysteine damage to endothelial cells. As subjects, they picked twenty-four healthy cigarette smokers in their late thirties. The smokers were randomly assigned to take a placebo or a 5 mg folic acid pill every day over a one-month period. Cigarette smoking increases homocysteine concentrations, endothelial dysfunction, and arterial stiffening. Homocysteine per se induces endothelial dysfunction and arterial stiffening, and might at least partly account for the vascular abnormalities observed in smokers. At the end of the short study, the researchers reported reduced homocysteine levels, enhanced arterial dilation (a sign of improved endothelial function), and lowered blood pressure among the supplemented smokers. "Thus, a simple, nontoxic, and relatively inexpensive vitamin intervention might be useful in primary cardiovascular prevention in this high-risk group," they said.

Three large recent studies have failed to find that the use of B vitamins to lower the homocysteine level has particular effectiveness for high-risk patients with advanced CVD or for those who have already experienced heart attacks. In these studies, many patients were taking strong medications that may have overshadowed specific B vitamin benefits. The evidence suggests that homocysteine is important in disease genesis—as an initiating factor—that acts over a period of many years. Thus, preventing elevated homocysteine should be the goal.

"It is essential to lower homocysteine to prevent the disease," says McCully. "And B-complex vitamins are critical for that. Once the atherosclerosis process is well advanced, homocysteine may no longer play a critical role. In the studies published so far, controlling the homocysteine level once appreciable disease has developed does not have a detectable effect."

Our Recommendations

Whether or not you have heart disease, we strongly advocate the whole range of B-complex vitamins, not just one or two. If you concentrate on just one, you may cause a relative deficiency in other B factors. For general prevention, a good multivitamin contains enough of the B vitamins.

If you have elevated homocysteine, take extra folic acid in milligram dosages (such as 1 to 5 mg), about 40 mg of B-6, and 200 mcg of B-12. Repeat the test for your homocysteine level two months after you start on a supplement program. If still high, add N-acetylcysteine, an excellent antioxidant, at 500 mg per day. Stomach acid is needed to liberate B vitamins from food. If you take an acid-suppressing drug, you may need additional B vitamins.

High intake of folic acid also helps the body convert L-arginine to nitric oxide (see the discussion earlier in this chapter on L-arginine). In the 1940s and 1950s, studies were done in which people were treated with huge amounts of folic acid, in the area of 50 mg, and their angina and claudication improved. The researchers hypothesized that folic acid opened up collateral vascularization. We now know that folic acid stimulates nitric oxide synthase, the enzyme that produces nitric oxide from L-arginine. So we are liberal with our folic acid recommendations. Five milligrams may do a lot more than just lower homocysteine. Work closely with your doctor if you would like to bump up your folic acid level.

A significant number of Canadians and Western Europeans have genetic defects that hinder their ability to utilize folic acid to bring down homocysteine. For these individuals, standard folic acid supplements have little or no effect. If you have tried different forms of folic acid with little success, try Metafolin, a patented, bioavailable form of folic acid (refer to the resources section in appendix A for information on how to order this product).

Cardiovascular considerations aside, the B vitamins are beneficial in the treatment of nervous problems, fatigue, and stress, and in the prevention of alcohol problems. Among the B vitamins, folic acid is the best deterrent against spina bifida, a disabling spinal birth defect. The B vitamins participate in the most important aspects of food metabolism, the production of energy, and immune function.

The only adverse effect we have seen from the B vitamins is constipation—from B-12—in a few patients. Generally, if you take too much vitamin B, your system excretes the excess. The B vitamins are water soluble.

If you notice your urine turns yellow after you start on a supplement program, the likely cause is vitamin B-2, which has a fluorescent yellow pigment. (The scientific term for B-2 is riboflavin, from the Latin word for yellow, *flavus*.) Don't be concerned. The body absorbs what it needs. The rest passes out through the urine.

Vitamin E

Vitamin E, a supplement with a long history of helping ailing hearts, has genuine merit in the treatment of active heart disease. We say this even though some recent controlled studies have been disappointing. Some of these studies, however, have been flawed in terms of design and type of vitamin used.

In 2004, vitamin E took a particular bashing when one statistical analysis of multiple studies suggested that high-dose vitamin E could result in a small increase in overall mortality. Although the analysis was misleading—the population of patients in the collected studies was already chronically sick and at high risk of dying—the publicity it generated shook many Americans' longstanding faith in vitamin E. Nearly a tenth of individuals polled in one national survey said they were unlikely to continue using the vitamin.

We are strong believers in vitamin E. But we have strong opinions on how and what you take.

First, taking more than 400 IU daily is unnecessary for individuals on a comprehensive supplement program. Second, high-dosage vitamin E by itself makes little sense. More is not better. One weakness of vitamin E is that it can become readily oxidized and contribute to the oxidation process in the blood. A group of Australian scientists at the Heart Research Institute in Sydney recently brought this problem to light. Under the direction of Roland Stocker, they made the fascinating discovery that vitamin E can itself become a highly energized and reactive compound when it scavenges free radicals. "Vitamin E can become a 'hot coal,' so to speak, potentially damaging other molecules unless it is brought back to a stable condition by a further partner in a chain which eventually terminates the process," says Stocker. Such partners are CoQ10 and vitamin C. They protect vitamin E and together make a powerful antioxidant front against CVD. In an experiment done with mice, it was shown that the combination of CoQ10 and vitamin E lowered oxidative stress in arterial walls, creating a more endothelial-friendly environment that decreased the CRP level and increased protection against inflammation.

Third, vitamin E is usually sold as a single compound called alpha-tocopherol. Optimally, it should be accompanied by gamma-tocopherol, a sibling compound with strong antioxidant properties. Too much alpha-tocopherol without gamma-tocopherol fails to eradicate certain types of dangerous free radicals such as the dangerous peroxynitrite radical.

But even used incorrectly, vitamin E has powerful effects, as many studies and vast clinical usage has demonstrated over the years:

- It decreases the two-year event rate of patients with newly diagnosed CVD by 50 percent.

- Vitamin E decreases the two-year heart attack rate by 75 percent in dialysis patients with known CVD.

- It decreases disease progression in men following bypass surgery.

- Together with aspirin in patients with TIA, vitamin E decreases the two-year stroke rate by 50 percent versus aspirin alone.

Our Recommendations

Read labels carefully. Don't just buy any vitamin E. You want 200 to 400 IU daily of natural vitamin E (D-alpha-tocopherol) in combination with the family of other vitamin E compounds, including gamma-tocopherol and tocotrienols. You can purchase these compounds together in one gel cap.

Avoid vitamin E with the designation of DL-alpha-tocopherol, which is a synthetic vitamin E. According to Margaret G. Traber, an expert on vitamin E at the Linus Pauling Institute, natural vitamin E has at least one and one half times greater absorption, delivery to tissues, and utilization than the synthetic form.

Vitamin E is fat soluble, so take it with food. You may even find enough vitamin E as part of a multisupplement. And although we recommend it, we don't single it out here as one of the frontline nutrients in our plaque-busting program of New Cardiology.

Garlic

In Bram Stoker's classic 1897 tale *Dracula*, the fair heroine Lucy uses a braid of garlic to fend off the blood-sucking count. Modern science has never gotten around to proving that garlic repels vampires, but it has repeatedly confirmed what healers throughout the ages have known: garlic is indeed nature's wonder drug.

Containing a veritable pharmacopoeia, including powerful sulfur and selenium compounds, garlic has been used for the prevention and treatment of diseases for thousands of years—from infections to heart conditions. One Egyptian medical papyrus, called the *Codex Elsers*, contained more than twenty medicinal formulas citing garlic as a cure for heart disease, worms, and tumors.

In more recent times, garlic has gained the reputation as a natural antibiotic. This germ-killing property is attributed to allicin, a sulfur compound that gives garlic its distinctive odor. Researchers have developed stabilized garlic compounds for use with supplements and found they have considerable promise against antibiotic-resistant bacterial strains.

Pathogens contribute to inflammation. Thus, garlic belongs in the armory of anti-CVD supplements. Another good, natural weapon against inflammation. Garlic is great in food, however, some of the garlic's medicinal potency is lost in cooking.

Selected Research

Studies show that garlic reduces multiple cardiovascular risk factors, including blood pressure, cholesterol, homocysteine, and platelet aggregation and adhesion, while stimulating nitric oxide generation in endothelial cells and raising HDL. Two medical reports in 2004 indicated that garlic can block the formation of plaque. In one study at Harbor-UCLA Medical Center in Torrance, California, researchers found that the addition of a garlic supplement significantly inhibited the progression of plaque calcification as measured by EBT imaging. One group of nine patients took an aged garlic extract supplement every day for a year while another group of ten subjects took a placebo. Disease progression in the placebo group averaged 22 percent, while plaque among the supplement group advanced only 7.5 percent.

Our Recommendations

For people with CVD, supplement with a minimum of 1,000 mg a day. Garlic also contributes to thinner blood. If you take Coumadin, you can still eat garlic, but don't use a garlic supplement.

Pomegranate Juice

Pomegranates have been cultivated for thousands of years, and because of their numerous seeds, they came to symbolize fertility, bounty, and immortality for various cultures and religions. The Spanish city of Granada takes its name from the Latin word for pomegranate, *granatum*.

Pomegranates are one of the richest sources of antioxidant flavonoids—healing nutrients found in plants. Recently, Israeli researchers have shown that these compounds slow the development of atherosclerotic plaque in mice and humans and help prevent LDL oxidation. In 2004, they reported on an experiment in which ten patients with severe carotid artery disease drank approximately 8 ounces of 100 percent pomegranate juice every day for one to three years. At the end of the study period, the researchers compared the juice drinkers to a matched group of patients who did not drink the juice, and they found a number of eye-opening differences:

- A 20 percent drop in systolic blood pressure in the juice drinkers

- A 19 percent reduction in oxidized LDL antibodies—a test for cholesterol oxidation activity—in the pomegranate juice drinkers

- A reduction in thickness of the carotid artery walls (30 percent, as compared to a 9 percent *increase* in the control group).

Throughout the trial, both groups had continued their usual medications, enabling the researchers to conclude that the flavonoids in pomegranates appear to offer some promising benefits for arterial disease.

In a 2005 study, pomegranate power was further confirmed by Italian researchers. They found that the juice significantly reduced the progression of arterial plaque in mice with high cholesterol. They also discovered that juice-bathed coronary artery endothelial cells produced more nitric oxide.

Larger human studies are certainly needed, but in the meantime filling up on pomegranate juice looks like a good idea for your heart. You can find the juice in health food stores and some grocery stores. Pomegranate supplements have already appeared on the market.

Our Recommendations

Drink a glass a day for therapeutic benefits. Brittle diabetics (patients supersensitive to sugar) should use caution and monitor their blood sugar. Always consume a healthy fat and/or protein snack with the juice if you're a diabetic.

Vitamin K-2

In 2006, both of us started working with MK7 (short for menaquinone-7), a form of vitamin K-2. The vitamin K you are most likely familiar with is K-1, found in green, leafy foods, such as kale, spinach, broccoli, and brussels sprouts. It is also available in supplement form.

However, K-2 is less abundant and harder to find. The highest concentration occurs in the fermented Japanese soy dish natto, which we highly recommend as "therapy food," as well as in fermented and curded cheese.

Both K-1 and K-2 are important for the health of bones and arterial tissue, but K-2 is clearly the more beneficial of the two nutrients. Recent research suggests that K-2 is more effective in slowing down the resorption of bone cells and increasing bone mineralization, which means stronger, healthier bones. It has also been shown to counteract arterial damage (atherosclerosis), which translates into better heart health.

Supplement Fundamentals

- Nutritional supplements work better together, in combination.
- When used alone, particularly in synthetic form or at the wrong dose, you don't get the maximum effect.
- When you stop taking supplements, you lose the benefits.
- Don't be confused by negative news reports. Educate yourself. Do some research. The Internet offers many authoritative and noncommercial resources on supplement research, including the Linus Pauling Institute (lpi.oregonstate.edu) and the U.S. government's National Library of Medicine (www.ncbi.nlm.nih.gov/entrez/).
- Vitamin A has come under scrutiny. Long-term use of vitamin A supplements—over twenty years—may increase the possibility of hip fracture. We don't recommend more than 5,000 units of pure vitamin A (retinyl palmitate) a day. We prefer natural carotenoids (such as beta-carotene), which the liver converts into vitamin A as needed. Beta-carotene supplementation cannot produce vitamin A overload.
- Patients often ask when to take supplements if they are also taking medication. Your best bet is to take them separately, an hour or two apart. Sometimes minerals will interfere with the absorption of a particular prescription medication. In some instances, absorption could be enhanced.
- Quality is king. Avoid inferior supplements and products with artificial dyes and sugar. If you have doubts, consult with a nutritionally oriented health professional who can recommend supplements for you.

In two studies with rabbits and rats, K-2 produced definite plaque reversal in their vessels. It appears that K-2 helps decalcify hard plaque formations. Similarly, a 2004 Dutch study analyzed the K-2 intake of nearly five thousand people and found a relationship between higher intake and reduced aortic calcification.

Low levels of vitamin K have long been associated with an increased incidence of osteoporotic fractures. Moreover, population-based analyses have consistently found widespread vitamin K deficiency. So K-2 appears to offer some intelligent, discriminating, and beneficial action: adding calcium in the bones, where it belongs, and removing it from the arteries, where it shouldn't be. That concept has us excited.

Our Recommendations

For both prevention and as part of a therapeutic program, we suggest eating natto two to three times a week. You can find it at Japanese grocers or health food stores. As for K-2 in supplement form, it is currently available only in low doses in a handful of bone formulas, not significant enough to have an effect against plaque. Dr. Sinatra has been developing a vitamin K-2 supplement, containing 150 mcg, which will be available in early 2007. We think that a daily intake level of 150 mcg will be needed. If you take Coumadin, you shouldn't take a vitamin K supplement, as it will neutralize Coumadin.

Chapter 7

Supplements

The ATP/Energy Boosters

A Medical Resurrection

One day in 1996, Dr. Sinatra received an urgent call from a man who pleaded with him to accept his mother as a transfer from another hospital. Louise was seventy-nine years old at the time and had been admitted to a community hospital with heart failure complicated by pneumonia.

Louise's son said she had been on a ventilator for several days, was getting powerful steroids and high concentrations of oxygen, but she was still failing. She went into kidney failure and her doctors said there was nothing more to do.

Louise's son was a biochemist and knowledgeable about the nutritional supplement CoQ10. He had asked the doctors at the hospital to place his mother on CoQ10. They refused. CoQ10 was not on their list of "approved formulas."

Louise's son brought in stacks of medical literature showing how CoQ10 could help patients with heart failure. The doctors would not review the information. Instead, they asked the family to end life support. The family refused. Louise's son then went to the hospital administrators. When he insisted on the CoQ10, they told him he was "interfering." The situation turned ugly. Lawyers became involved.

Dr. Sinatra told Louise's son that if his mother could be transferred to Manchester Memorial Hospital in Connecticut, where he could attend to her, he would make sure she received CoQ10, which was approved for use at the hospital.

Still, the transfer was risky in her weakened state. She would have to be transported in an ambulance and be "bag-breathed" for the journey of forty minutes or so—meaning a skilled medical technician would have to "breathe" her mechanically by hand the whole way.

Louise's son was quick to respond. The transfer was carried out. The elderly woman arrived semicomatose and respiratory dependent. She was placed on conventional pulmonary care similar to that she received at the previous hospital. The only change in her therapy was nutritional: 450 mg of CoQ10 given through a feeding tube daily, along with a multivitamin/mineral preparation and 1 gram of magnesium intravenously.

Although Dr. Sinatra had some hope for her, the other critical care doctors were extremely skeptical of using CoQ10 in this life-threatening case.

On the third day, she started to "wake up." After ten days, she was weaned off the ventilator. At two weeks, she was discharged to an extended care facility, sitting up in a wheelchair with only supplemental oxygen.

Dr. Sinatra then put Louise on a combined program of medications and broad nutritional supplement support, including 500 mg of CoQ10 daily. She followed the recommendations to the letter and lived for another seven years with a good quality of life.

This case was truly a medical resurrection and powerfully demonstrates the great lifesaving and life-extending potential of CoQ10. But the story is not unusual. Dr. Sinatra has personally treated many cases and has heard about many others in which people seemingly left for dead have been similarly resurrected by CoQ10.

Our heart failure readmission rate at hospitals is practically nil thanks to CoQ10 (coenzyme Q10), L-carnitine, D-ribose, and magnesium. These nutritional supplements nourish and support the mitochondria, the cellular power plants that generate ATP, the energy source for the primary biochemical reactions in the body. We covered magnesium in chapter 6. Now we turn our attention to CoQ10, L-carnitine, and D-ribose.

The cells of the heart muscle are loaded with mitochondria. And if they don't get enough of these raw materials—a result, for example, of inflammation and plaque that clog the arteries to the heart—the mitochondria and energy production suffer. When this occurs and when sections of the heart muscle die due to blocked arteries, we call the condition heart failure. The pump loses power.

How important is ATP? Joanne Ingwall, a professor of physiology at Harvard University and an expert on energy metabolism of the heart, informs us that every event in the myocyte (heart cell) directly or indirectly requires ATP. In her book *ATP and the Heart*, she writes that heart cells need ATP to maintain a normal heart rate, pump blood, and support increased work, as well as to grow, repair themselves, and survive. "The requirement for ATP is absolute."

Unfortunately, we cannot put ATP into a supplement, give it to people with a compromised heart muscle, and see instant rejuvenation. But we can assist the body to make ATP naturally. We do this routinely for our patients—we call it metabolic cardiology—with the simple addition of a few nutritional supplements.

Cardiac muscle cells work nonstop to fuel an organ that pumps sixty to a hundred times a minute, twenty-four hours a day, for years and years. This constant energy demand makes the heart especially vulnerable to even subtle deficiencies of the raw materials contributing to ATP generation. In metabolic cardiology, we encourage the heart's enzymatic energy reactions in a preferential direction as opposed to the pharmaceutical approach that blocks enzymatic reactions. We do it with CoQ10, L-carnitine, and D-ribose. They feed the enzymatic production of ATP in the mitochondria.

Angina patients have gone beyond a critical metabolic threshold. They have burned off their CoQ10 and L-carnitine and ATP precursor pool. The more frequent and more severe the angina, the lower the content of these nutrients in the heart. Each episode depletes more of them, leaving the heart muscle without enough ATP to operate normally. The worse shape the heart is in, the more urgent the need to supplement.

These supplements are also great medicine for patients with a history of heart failure, severe high blood pressure, and heart attack—situations in which the heart works overtime. Even healthy athletes benefit because their hearts work harder than nature intended.

Coenzyme Q10 (CoQ10)

More than four thousand scientific studies and twelve international conferences have distinguished CoQ10 as a healing superstar and lifesaver. It does all these things:

- Prevents disease and slows down the aging process
- Helps patients with all forms of heart disease
- Reduces mild to moderate hypertension
- Generates energy, strength, and vitality, even for older people
- Fortifies the immune system against illness, including cancer
- Counteracts the adverse effects of cholesterol-lowering drugs (statins)
- Improves nervous system and brain disorders
- Protects against gum disease, a condition affecting most adults

CoQ10 is a fat-soluble vitamin. Despite strong scientific evidence for CoQ10's benefits, most doctors either haven't heard of CoQ10 or ignore its importance. To us this represents a major tragedy, because simply putting patients on a risk-free CoQ10 supplement pays off with health, energy, and therapeutic dividends.

Since the 1970s, scientists throughout the world have reported on the healing impact of CoQ10, primarily on cardiovascular conditions. But during the last decade, research has expanded dynamically into many age-related neurodegenerative diseases, such as Alzheimer's disease, Parkinson's disease, and Lou Gehrig's disease, and it has focused attention on mitochondrial involvement. As researchers probe deeper into the mitochondrial and bioenergetic basis of disease and the aging process itself, CoQ10 figures to keep gaining importance. Rolf Luft, of the Karolinska Hospital in Sweden, a pioneer in mitochondrial medicine, has observed that even a relatively small deficiency of CoQ10 may be a key factor in the development of many disorders.

Cells make energy from oxygen and the sugars and fatty acids from food. These raw materials pass through cell membranes and are dispatched to the mitochondria, where the raw materials are processed by enzymes to produce ATP. Electrons extracted from the food are used to make ATP. CoQ10 molecules carry out a critical role in this process by shuttling electrons back and forth between enzymes. In 1978, the British biochemist Peter Mitchell won the Nobel Prize in chemistry for describing this complicated and exquisite step in cellular energy production.

This activity is the primary function of CoQ10 in the body, according to the biochemist Karl Folkers, the world's leading authority on CoQ10 until his death in 1997. For nearly forty years, Folkers passionately conducted and encouraged CoQ10 research. In 1972, as the director of the Institute for Biomedical Research at the University of Texas at Austin, his investigations led to the discovery of CoQ10 deficiency in heart disease. This original research inspired numerous other studies showing major therapeutic benefits for supplemented heart patients. For his years of outstanding research, Folkers was honored with the Presidential Science Award by President George H. W. Bush in 1990.

Multiple studies have confirmed widespread CoQ10 deficiency among CVD patients. One study found deficiencies in three-fourths of 132 patients undergoing heart surgery. The most serious deficits occur among patients with weak hearts, suffering from conditions such as cardiomyopathy or heart failure. Ailing hearts, young and old alike, can be helped with CoQ10. It works for teenagers with cardiomyopathy, baby boomers with blocked arteries, and octogenarians with failing hearts.

In cardiomyopathy, the heart muscle becomes inflamed and dilated and doesn't pump well. It enlarges to pump more blood. When the heart can't pump enough blood, the condition is called heart failure. This life-threatening situation can also result from narrowed arteries, a past heart attack with scarring of the heart muscle, high blood pressure, a congenital heart defect (present at birth), or heart valve dysfunction.

With heart failure, swelling (edema) often results, typically in the legs and ankles. Fluid builds up in the lungs and interferes with breathing, causing shortness of breath. The condition also impairs the kidneys' ability to dispose of sodium and water. Poor blood flow to the muscles leads to fatigue and a low threshold for exertion.

Drugs, including diuretics, are the standard treatment. When that fails, a patient may become a candidate for a heart transplant.

The Miracle Supplement

In the early 1980s, Folkers collaborated with Per Langsjoen, of the Scott and White Clinic in Temple, Texas, in the first well-controlled cardiomyopathy study of CoQ10. The effect of the supplement on nineteen patients, all of whom were expected to die of heart failure, was astounding. They made an "extraordinary clinical improvement," the researchers said. Heart size decreased and blood pumping improved, regardless of the form of cardiomyopathy.

Subsequent research involving thousands of CVD patients has produced similar results: significant improvements in quality of life and longer survival. These benefits apply not just to cardiomyopathy and heart failure but to angina, coronary artery disease, heart attack, and recovery from heart surgery.

The cardiologist Peter Langsjoen, of Tyler, Texas, has participated in CoQ10 studies since the early 1980s. First with his cardiologist father, Per, who passed away in 1993, and subsequently in his own private practice, Langsjoen has logged more clinical usage of CoQ10 than any other U.S. doctor.

"It's the backbone of my cardiac practice, and I find it unthinkable to practice medicine without it," said Langsjoen. "Based on more than ten thousand patients, I can unequivocally say it does a great deal of good for many people without any side effects. Using CoQ10 is like watering a dry plant. It's that remarkable. The sicker the patient, the more striking the results. In eighty percent of my patients, I see improvement in four weeks, with maximum improvement in six to twelve months, when they reach a plateau and have no additional cardiovascular benefits. As their heart function improves, we have to decrease their medicines."

CoQ10's most powerful therapeutic application is for any impairment in heart muscle function because the heart uses such a huge amount of energy. That's where you see the dramatic lifesaving changes.

"This includes ischemic [lack of oxygen] conditions, such as coronary artery disease, because the CoQ10 energizes the viable cells left in the heart muscle," says Langsjoen.

Indeed, CoQ10 offers impressive benefits for atherosclerosis and CAD by reenergizing heart cells, including cells in trouble that may either die or struggle to live. This is part of CoQ10's magic. It can rejuvenate those cells.

Let's say the heart muscle is getting poor blood flow, just enough to maintain life. CoQ10 enables it to function better with whatever limited flow it receives. As a result, a patient will have less chest pain—in fact, quite a bit less—not because the arteries are being opened but because of better energy production in the low-flow regions of the muscle. CoQ10 permits more ATP generation from available oxygen.

"CoQ10 is a huge heart supplement," said Langsjoen.

After thirty plus years of collectively using this miracle nutrient, we unequivocally say amen. This supplement has worked miracles for many of our patients.

Bypass the Transplant?

In 1994, the largest study of CoQ10 and heart failure was reported in the journal *Molecular Aspects of Medicine*. Researchers at different Italian medical centers gave more than twenty-five hundred patients 50 to 150 mg of CoQ10 daily for three months. The majority took 100 mg.

Improved quality of life was reported by 78 percent of the patients. Fifty-four percent attained significant improvement in at least three clinical signs that included general fluid retention, pulmonary fluid retention, heart palpitations, liver enlargement, and shortness of breath.

Such positive outcomes, along with many documented clinical reports, prompted Folkers to make a strong appeal for the use of CoQ10 among individuals considering a heart transplant. Writing in the journal *Biochemical and Biophysical Research Communications*, Folkers argued that research has clearly "established the efficacy and safety of CoQ10 to treat patients in heart failure. In the U.S., about 20,000 patients under sixty-five years are eligible for transplants, but donors number less than ⅒th of those eligible, and there are many more such patients over sixty-five, both eligible and ineligible."

In the report, Folkers, along with both Langsjoens, described eleven transplant cases treated with CoQ10. "After CoQ10, all improved," they said. "Some patients required no conventional drugs and had no limitation in lifestyle." One of the cases involved a sixty-four-year-old African American male with a failing heart and inoperable coronary disease. After six months, he had improved to the point where he had "no limitation whatsoever on his activities." Many such dramatically positive cases like this, combined with the absence of side effects, "justify treating patients in failure . . . with CoQ10," the researchers said.

Heart failure has been strongly correlated with low blood and tissue levels of CoQ10. The more severe the degree of disease, the greater the CoQ10 deficiency. This finding led Folkers to propose that the actual molecular cause of cardiac failure may be a "dominant deficiency" of CoQ10. "Even if you treat a patient with a conventional drug, the CoQ10 deficiency still remains," he said. "No cardiovascular drug can do for the human body what CoQ10 can do."

Antioxidant Supreme

Coenzyme Q10 rates as one of the most powerful antioxidants known. First and foremost, it protects the mitochondria, where tremendous amounts of free radicals are produced in the cellular generation of energy. CoQ10 feeds the energy process but also nips in the bud the most powerful oxidative reactions that can harm the body.

In addition, CoQ10 travels through the bloodstream, circulating with other antioxidants such as vitamin E to help prevent oxidation of cholesterol. It also protects vitamin E itself from free radical destruction, a protective relationship just recently discovered.

In a 2004 study in the *American Journal of Clinical Nutrition*, an animal (baboon) model showed that CoQ10 and vitamin E together reduced CRP, the potent inflammatory marker and mediator of CAD.

It turns out that CoQ10 molecules in the bloodstream are actually transported by LDL cholesterol. CoQ10 protects LDL from oxidation.

In a 1992 study on healthy young adults, investigators found CoQ10 generated a "remarkable resistance" of LDL to oxidative damage. Too much oxidized LDL leads to the formation of plaque. One study published in the *Proceedings of the National Academy of Sciences USA* suggests that CoQ10 may, in fact, be far more effective than other antioxidants in blocking LDL oxidation.

Animal studies demonstrate that CoQ10 supplementation gives significant protections against arterial plaque, even when animals are fed diets designed to raise the level of cholesterol and other fats in their bodies. Thus, CoQ10's antioxidant power benefits both the heart and the blood vessels that supply it.

CoQ10, especially in the presence of gamma-tocopherol (a vitamin E compound), helps to neutralize the damaging effects of peroxynitrite, a particularly damaging free radical that is considered toxic to endothelial and smooth muscle arterial cells. This connection suggests that CoQ10 reduces oxidative stress within the arterial wall.

CoQ10 and Heart Attack

In 1998, Indian researchers reported on the ability of CoQ10 to provide "rapid protective effects" in acute heart attack patients if administered within three days of the onset of symptoms. In one experiment, they treated 144 patients conventionally, except 73 were randomly selected to take 100 mg of CoQ10 daily for a month. The results: CoQ10 patients fared significantly better, with less heart failure, arrhythmias, and second heart attacks:

	CoQ10 Group	*Non-CoQ10 Group*
FOUR WEEKS AFTER TREATMENT		
Adverse events	15 percent	32 percent
ONE YEAR AFTER TREATMENT		
Adverse events	25 percent	48 percent
Death rate	11 percent	20 percent

CoQ10 and Heart Surgery

A 1993 study at St. Vincent Indianapolis Hospital demonstrated the dramatic benefits of CoQ10 on ejection fraction, heart muscle ATP content, and outcome in elderly patients scheduled for high-risk bypass surgery. In this experiment, ten out of twenty patients were randomly selected to take 100 mg of CoQ10 daily for two weeks before surgery and for a month afterward.

Bypass surgery generates free radicals and interferes with ATP metabolism. Heart muscle tissue samples obtained at the start of surgery revealed 50 percent more CoQ10 and ATP in the supplemented patients. After the study, the researchers reported the following differences among patients:

	CoQ10 Patients	Non-CoQ10 Patients
Heart muscle ATP level	Higher than baseline	Plummeted
Heart muscle CoQ10 level	Higher than baseline	Plummeted
Immediate postbypass ejection fraction average	40 percent	20 percent
Recovery average	3–5 days	15–30 days
Deaths	0	2
Requirement for kidney dialysis	0	3

Australian cardiologists at the Alfred Hospital Cardiac Surgical Research Unit in Melbourne have repeatedly found that supplementation with CoQ10 prior to heart surgery accelerates recovery and protects against surgical complications. In their latest study, 122 patients were randomly selected to take either CoQ10 or an inert placebo pill for one week before elective coronary artery bypass graft surgery. The amount of CoQ10 used was 300 mg a day.

Following surgery, the CoQ10 patients developed superior ATP production, better heart muscle contraction, less heart muscle damage, and spent less time recovering in the hospital.

"If a surgeon would like his heart patients to recover better and have a stronger heart muscle, CoQ10 supplementation should be a real option to use," said Franklin Rosenfeldt, head of the research unit.

More than half a million bypass surgeries are performed in the United States each year. They involve increasingly older patients and an increasing percentage of repeat operations. As a result, injury, death, and cost have risen substantially. Multiple studies show that pretreatment with CoQ10 improves the postoperative status of not just bypass patients but also heart valve replacement patients. Hopefully, cardiologists will recognize the value that a simple supplementation program can contribute to surgical outcomes.

An Anti-CoQ10 Bias?

Dr. Roberts: In Toledo, where I practice, patients who undergo bypass surgery at one major hospital are not permitted to take CoQ10. I've sent packages of medical journal articles to the hospital's pharmacy and therapeutics committee. I've had no response. I doubt they even read the papers. Medical arrogance like this costs lives. My patients know about the CoQ10 studies. I've heard that some sneak their CoQ10 into the hospital. They don't want to die from arrogance.

CoQ10 and High Blood Pressure

As far back as 1976, researchers noted that CoQ10 decreases blood pressure in patients with established hypertension. Over the years, the evidence has continued to grow and now points to CoQ10 deficiency as a *cause* of high blood pressure in some people.

Heart muscle cells, as we know, are packed with mitochondria and utilize a lot of CoQ10. In any disease that affects heart muscle function, whether CAD, diabetes, or mitral valve disease, the first change that occurs is a stiffening and thickening of the heart muscle. This phenomenon may very well be the result of a CoQ10 deficiency. The stiffening means the heart has to work harder in order to fill its chambers with blood and then pump it out again. In response, the body produces adrenaline, the stress hormone. It raises the heart rate and improves the filling and pumping action. However, on a continual basis, the increased adrenaline causes a general constriction of the blood vessels, which means that higher (more) blood pressure is required to push the blood through narrowed arteries.

To date, about a dozen studies, most of them small, have shown improvement in heart muscle function and gradual lowering of blood pressure with CoQ10. As blood pressure gradually normalizes, patients may often start reducing their medication. They report improvement in their quality of life and vigor. Obviously, CoQ10 exerts an energizing effect, but improvement also relates to taking less medication.

CoQ10 and Diabetes

Medical studies reveal a deficiency of CoQ10 in diabetic patients. In one study, 120 mg per day of CoQ10 given to thirty-nine patients with diabetes resulted in a reduction of blood sugar levels by 20 to 30 percent. This effect is not well known. Clearly, we need more research to clarify a potential role for CoQ10, but by energizing cells and making tissues work more efficiently, we change the fundamental cellular chemistry of everything in a positive direction.

CoQ10 and Gum Disease

A significant relationship exists between gum disease and chronic inflammation. As the numbers and activity of multiple microbes—bacteria, spirochetes, and viruses—build up around teeth and gums, they create an inflammatory mode throughout the body. This, in turn, has been found to be a risk factor for CVD.

In the 1970s, researchers in Europe and Japan found that many patients with diseased gums were deficient in CoQ10. Further studies showed that supplementation had a marked therapeutic effect. In one double-blind clinical experiment over a three-week period, patients were randomly given either a placebo pill or CoQ10. The eight patients on CoQ10 all improved significantly: less bleeding, pain, and swelling. They healed faster. Patients taking placebo pills showed no improvement. The researchers commented that the results seen after three weeks of supplementation normally take six months with standard treatment.

CoQ10 Deficiency

Nature designed our cells to make CoQ10 from different vitamins, minerals, and amino acids. A deficiency of any of these nutrients harms CoQ10 production, notably folic acid; vitamins C, B-12, B-6, and pantothenic acid (B-5); and certain minerals. Thus, poor diet negatively impacts your CoQ10 level. So does the aging process, an overactive thyroid, antidepressants, and gum disease. Vegetarians tend to have lower levels. Athletes, or individuals involved in continual high-intensity exercise, also register low on the CoQ10 scale, most probably the result of a free radical torrent caused by the massive metabolic demands of overworking muscles.

It's clear to see why CoQ10 deficiency is quite common, yet harder to understand why it is so overlooked. Research indicates that if the CoQ10 level in your body drops by 25 percent, your organs may become deficient and functionally impaired. At 75 percent, serious tissue damage and even death may occur. Sophisticated diagnostic studies tell us that blood and heart tissue levels are quite low in cases of advanced heart failure.

Another major cause of depletion: statin drugs prescribed to lower cholesterol. They interfere with the internal production of CoQ10. If you take a statin drug regularly and start experiencing muscle pain or weakness, your body is telling you that CoQ10 has been depleted to the point of causing symptoms. Given the evidence, we consider it neglectful for doctors to prescribe statin drugs without a CoQ10 supplement.

Typical signs of CoQ10 depletion from statin usage include aches and pains, fatigue, malaise, sore muscles, weakness, the feeling of a low-grade flu, and shorter breath with exertion. Forgetfulness and mental confusion may develop as well. Signs are deceiving. They usually develop over time. Gradually you start feeling worse and just don't attribute it to a medication you started last month or even a year or two before.

In 2001, the International CoQ10 Association attempted to bring this issue to the attention of the FDA. In a letter signed by fourteen scientists and clinicians in seven countries, the group pointed out that muscle destruction and fatigue linked to statins may be a direct result of CoQ10 depletion. The scientists also noted that although statin therapy has benefits, its long-term benefits against heart disease may be blunted due to CoQ10 loss. The association urged the agency to study "whether the clinical use of statins can be made safer and possibly more effective by the addition of CoQ10." It urged an investigation in order "to prevent further developments of what have already been serious medical consequences." The association never received a reply from the FDA.

The Canadian government, however, has taken a first step, requiring that statins sold in Canada carry a warning label stating that CoQ10 depletion can lead to impaired cardiac functioning in patients with heart failure.

Word is getting out. At the American College of Cardiology's 2005 scientific conference, doctors learned of a simple thirty-day trial with CoQ10 that significantly reduced statin-induced muscle pain. Another study demonstrated that statin therapy leads to diastolic dysfunction, our term for increased stiffness of the heart muscle, which plays a role in shortness of breath and heart failure (we discussed this in the statin section of chapter 5). Concomitant CoQ10 supplementation resolved the problem. The researchers said they were trying to address a very important clinical question—that is, to capture the benefits of statin therapy without producing complications due to statin-induced CoQ10 depletion.

Issues about Supplement Dosage and Form

Pure CoQ10—bioidentical to what your body produces—is manufactured through a fermentation process from yeast. The Kaneka Corporation of Japan is the world leader in this technology and also the largest supplier of CoQ10 for supplement usage. Asahi and Mitsubishi are other major producers. These three Japanese suppliers provide the highest quality. They ship the raw material in powder form to supplement companies around the world. Prior to the mid-1990s, these companies sold their CoQ10 in the form of capsule-filled powder, the form that researchers first used.

Animal and cell culture studies show that supplementation increases both tissue and mitochondrial levels of CoQ10. If sufficient CoQ10 can reach the bloodstream, our cells will readily take it in. The problem with taking CoQ10 by mouth is that the substance is a big molecule and doesn't absorb well in the dry powder capsule form. Researchers and clinicians needed to use larger dosages in order to obtain solid therapeutic results and had to use even more for advanced conditions. Then the good results came. Studies that failed to show results were not a consequence of CoQ10 ineffectiveness but rather the failure of researchers to use enough CoQ10.

A Dosage "Mistake" That Saved the Day

The following case history from Dr. Sinatra's patient file makes the dosage point very clear.

Lucy first developed symptoms of heart failure when she was sixty.

Her condition was brought on by longstanding high blood pressure that weakened her left ventricle. By age sixty-seven, she was congested with fluid in her lungs (pulmonary edema). Her ejection fraction was only 35 percent. (The normal range is 50 to 70 percent.) After a second episode of pulmonary edema, a cardiac catheterization (angiogram) showed an enlarged, stretched, and weakened left ventricle and normal coronary arteries. She was treated by another physician with standard medications.

Lucy's health progressively went downhill. By the time she consulted with Dr. Sinatra in 1996, she was almost eighty and struggling for every breath. She weighed only 77 pounds and suffered from severe weakness and weight loss, the symptoms of end-stage cardiac cachexia—a general physical wasting and malnutrition associated with chronic disease.

Her echocardiogram showed a leaky valve and an ejection fraction now of only 15 percent, barely enough to support a bed-to-chair lifestyle. Dr. Sinatra prescribed 30 mg of CoQ10 three times a day (90 mg/day), at the time a standard therapeutic dosage. Despite the supplement, she developed marked edema, ascites (a collection of fluids in body cavities, especially the abdomen), and severe fatigue. Her breathing became so labored that she required two lung taps to withdraw the excess fluid from her chest. Lucy remained homebound, slowly dying.

But then Lucy accidentally started taking 300 mg of CoQ10 daily—more than triple her customary dosage. Her son had mistakenly purchased 100 mg capsules instead of the usual 30 mg supplements. Four weeks later, Lucy called to say she was feeling better every day. She was advised to continue the 300 mg dosage.

Three months later, Lucy was significantly active and mobile. A repeat echocardiogram showed her ejection fraction now at 20 percent—a rise of one-third. An ultrasound of her heart indicated reduced valve leakage.

A year after she began taking CoQ10 supplements and eight months after her dosage "mistake," Lucy was out shopping and visiting relatives. She became so active, in fact, that she fell down and fractured her hip! Previously considered a high surgical risk, she underwent a successful hip replacement operation. Her CoQ10 blood level was 4.8 µg/ml on 300 mg of CoQ10 daily, an ideal level for her severe cardiac condition. We have learned over the years that blood levels must be greater than 3.5 µg/ml to make a difference in severely compromised patients like Lucy.

Improved CoQ10 Forms

In recent years, supplement companies have developed improved delivery systems that enhance CoQ10 uptake and utilization by the cells. At the time of the writing of this book, maximum bioavailability appears to be achieved by a hydrosoluble processing technology that enhances CoQ10 absorption in both water and fat so that it is readily picked up in the bloodstream. Next best are oil-based soft-gel supplements in which the CoQ10 is dissolved in an oil medium such as soybean. Recently, a dextrose compound called cyclodextrin has been complexed with CoQ10 to improve the absorption of the powder-in-capsule supplements.

Form is a principal consideration when reading the science or deciding which supplement to choose. Form determines dosage.

The medical literature contains multiple studies showing the positive effects of CoQ10 supplementation for compromised cardiac patients. The usual recommended dosage: 100 to 200 mg daily. But, as the case of Lucy clearly teaches us, some patients may not respond to such doses. They need more. When we have critically ill patients like Lucy, we ask ourselves several questions when considering dosage:

- Will the dosage sufficiently raise a patient's CoQ10 blood level?

- Does the CoQ10 supplement the patient takes actually deliver the amount stated on the label? Is it a form readily absorbed?

- How do I know the patient's level of CoQ10 without drawing blood levels?

An adequate CoQ10 dosage typically yields symptom improvement. Lack of improvement suggests the need for higher dosage. Increase the dosage and maintain it over time. More patients can recapture their quality of life with this aggressive approach. The sickest patients stand to gain the most from high dosages.

We encounter many new patients taking large doses of CoQ10 but without significant therapeutic effects. Testing frequently determines they even have a low or a normal blood level of CoQ10 despite the fact they take 200 to 400 mg daily. This can indicate one of two things:

1. The patient doesn't absorb the supplement.

2. The product may be at fault. Either it doesn't contain enough pure CoQ10, or its particular form has inferior bioavailability or contains filler compounds that interfere with absorption. Beware of "bargain" CoQ10 supplements. They may contain far less CoQ10

in the product than what the label claims, and they are often poorly absorbed.

Since adequate blood levels and bioavailability of CoQ10 are essential to treating very sick people, we offer some additional information designed to make your use of this remarkable supplement the most beneficial for you. The differences in CoQ10 forms have created confusion not just among consumers and patients but among physicians as well.

CoQ10 Blood-Level Research

After you swallow a pill, CoQ10 travels the same pathway of intestinal absorption as other fats we consume. Among the factors affecting this process are particle size, degree of solubility (that is, dissolvability), and the type of food eaten with the supplement. Absorption is helped, for instance, by taking the supplement with a meal containing some fat, which provides a medium for the CoQ10 to mix with.

Commercially available CoQ10 supplements come in different forms: CoQ10 dissolved in oil-filled soft-gel capsules (the most common), tablets, chew tabs, wafers, and the original powder-filled hard-shell capsules. A few published reports have compared the absorption or bioavailability of CoQ10 products. In one of them, researchers compared the bioavailability of three commercially available solubilized (CoQ10 dissolved in oil) soft gels against each other and against a baseline reference of one nonsolubilized capsule (powder) preparation. Bioavailability was measured by how quickly the CoQ10 was absorbed into the blood and how the blood level was affected following administration. Each subject in this test received a single 180 mg dose of a test CoQ10 product. The blood level was tested at set intervals. After a two-week washout period (no supplementation), another CoQ10 product was given to the same individuals. And then again a third product was administered. This type of study is called a crossover study. The design allows researchers to see how each test subject reacts to a given preparation.

Powder-filled capsules fared poorly in the study. However, each of the fully solubilized preparations was quickly absorbed. Blood levels of CoQ10 reached their peak in approximately six hours following administration and remained elevated for six days.

Dr. Sinatra was involved as an investigator in two other studies comparing relative bioavailability of commercially available products, including an oil suspension in a soft-gel capsule, powder-filled capsule, tablet, and hydrosoluble soft-gel capsule (Q-Gel). Each of the studies involved twenty-four healthy adult volunteers. The hydrosolubilized form raised the CoQ10 blood level the highest, reaching a therapeutic range above a desired 2.5 µg/ml level within three to four weeks. Further increases developed as time went on.

The most recent bioavailability study on CoQ10 preparations was reported in 2004 in the *New Zealand Medical Journal*. The study was motivated out of concern about CoQ10 depletion among more than a hundred thousand patients taking statins in New Zealand. The researchers independently tested seven different blends of CoQ10 without the knowledge of any of the manufacturers. Again, hydrosoluble CoQ10 (Q-Gel) scored significantly higher than any other form of CoQ10 supplement—in this case, 300 percent better than the average of the other products.

Although an optimal CoQ10 dosage is not yet known for every disease situation, researchers agree that blood levels of 2.5 µg/ml and preferably 3.5 µg/ml are required for a therapeutic impact on severely diseased hearts. Therefore, physicians employing CoQ10 as a therapeutic supplement should determine bioavailability through blood testing. Regardless of the brand and form of CoQ10 you use, the blood level is the bottom line.

Our Recommendations

We use the hydrosoluble CoQ10 in our practices and take it ourselves. There are multiple brands widely available that use hydrosoluble technology. Look for Q-Gel somewhere on the label.

The dosage recommendations listed below are for standard forms of CoQ10, not hydrosoluble. If you choose a hydrosoluble product—our preference—take about one-half the dosages given here. Thus, a 120 mg dosage of standard CoQ10 translates to 60 mg of Q-Gel.

- 60 to 120 mg as a preventive for cardiovascular or periodontal disease
- 180 to 360 mg for the treatment of angina pectoris, cardiac arrhythmia, high blood pressure, and moderate gum disease and for patients taking statin drugs
- 300 to 360 mg for mild to moderate heart failure
- 360 to 600 mg for severe heart failure and dilated cardiomyopathy
- 600 to 1,200 mg for an improvement in quality of life in Parkinson's disease

For maximum absorption, take CoQ10 with meals. If higher dosages are needed, divide the CoQ10 over two or more meals a day.

Once a therapeutic effect occurs—such as improved well-being, lowered blood pressure, better breathing, and healthier gums—adjust down to a maintenance dosage. For many cardiac conditions, especially heart failure and cardiomyopathy, the higher therapeutic dosage must be maintained or symptoms will return. Patients well maintained on one particular form of CoQ10 might have a return of symptoms if they change brand or dosage.

As noted, we test our patients to determine CoQ10 blood level. The test tells us if we are getting absorption and a blood level high enough to achieve the desired therapeutic objective. We list the targeted therapeutic blood levels in chapter 12. Ask your doctor to perform the CoQ10 blood-level test to ensure that your dosage is effective.

Do-It-Yourself Absorption Test

How can you readily tell if you are absorbing your CoQ10 supplement well? Try this simple test:

Take your supplement—whether it's a powder-filled capsule, soft gel, or wafer—and empty the contents into a clear glass of very warm water.

Now watch what happens.

If the contents go into a colloidal suspension after twenty minutes or so, spreading evenly and uniformly throughout the water, you've got a product that dissolves well and should be amply available to the cells in your body.

If, however, it creates an oily slick on the surface of the water or does anything but suspend, then it's not optimally crossing the cell membranes.

Precautions

The two of us have prescribed CoQ10 collectively for more than two decades. We have not seen any significant adverse reactions despite the fact that many of our patients take hundreds of milligrams a day. Although we don't know of any absolute contraindications to CoQ10, we do not recommend it for healthy pregnant women, nursing mothers, newborns, or very young children. There is not enough data on its use in these populations. However, in pregnant or nursing mothers with heart disease, we have used CoQ10 with no adverse effects.

Not only statins but beta blockers can inhibit CoQ10 activity in the body. This may explain why some patients with heart failure worsen on beta blockers. CoQ10 supplementation reduces beta blocker–induced fatigue. We have used CoQ10 in conjunction with beta blockers, especially for the treatment of high blood pressure, arrhythmia, and angina. The combination works very well.

Doctors should carefully monitor PT/INR in patients using Coumadin, especially if they feel CoQ10 therapy is also indicated. Careful monitoring can allow the successful therapeutic use of both. One need not exclude the other. We have used this combination safely in hundreds of our patients over the years. We have had to adjust the Coumadin level only on rare occasions.

L-carnitine

The oxygen-starved hearts of patients with both coronary artery disease and heart failure struggle constantly to pump hard enough to keep the blood moving forward. They are the most compromised of all people with CVD. The more advanced the disease, the less oxygen available and the weaker the heart becomes. Increasingly we see blood congestion backing up into the lungs and tissues.

We have had excellent results using CoQ10 for these patients. About 85 percent respond, but 15 percent still remain severely limited despite good CoQ10 blood levels. We've been happy to discover that supplementation with the amino acid L-carnitine, along with CoQ10, has helped relieve the symptoms of many patients in this predicament. Research suggests that L-carnitine and CoQ10 work synergistically to raise ATP production, and our experience validates this idea. The addition of L-carnitine provides a big boost in energy. When these refractory patients return for office follow-ups with better color, less labored breathing, and less difficulty with exertion, it's a cardiologist's dream come true.

Like CoQ10, L-carnitine belongs to a group of nutrients similar to many vitamins in that they are obtained from the diet through food sources and also made in the body. L-carnitine performs two major functions inside the mitochondria:

1. L-carnitine transports fatty acids to be oxidized to make ATP. It alone does this essential shuttling job, so the body needs a lot of it. The normal heart derives 60 to 70 percent of its fuel from fat, so for

anyone with heart disease, efficient fat delivery to the mitochondria is a must. Without L-carnitine, fatty acids cannot be transported to the inner mitochondrial membrane where ATP production occurs. This core process that also involves CoQ10 depends on the quantity of available L-carnitine. An increased concentration accelerates energy metabolism. Low concentration impairs it.

2. L-carnitine also transports waste material out of the mitochondria, such as toxic metabolites that could otherwise disturb the burning of fats and cause disruption inside cells.

L-carnitine is burned up in the heart under strain. Just as with CoQ10, the more advanced the heart disease, the lower the L-carnitine concentration present and the greater the need for it. Similarly, the more advanced the heart disease, the more responsive the patient to supplementation.

L-carnitine comes from two amino acids: lysine and methionine. Your body mixes these aminos with niacin, vitamin B-6, and vitamin C to form L-carnitine. Although deficiency is rare in healthy, well-nourished people consuming adequate protein, many individuals appear to have some deficiency.

Pure vegetarians miss out on common dietary sources of L-carnitine, just as they do with CoQ10. We see many vegetarians with low blood levels of both. The word *carnitine* comes from the Latin word *carnis*, meaning flesh or meat. The highest quantities of L-carnitine are found in mutton from older sheep, followed by lamb, beef, other red meat, and pork. The least amount is found in plant food. Many vegetarians fail to get enough L-carnitine in their diet and may also lack the methionine and lysine needed to synthesize it in their bodies.

Other reasons for L-carnitine deficiencies include genetic defects; aging; cofactor deficiencies of vitamin B-6, folic acid, iron, niacin, and especially vitamin C; liver or kidney disease; and the use of certain medications, particularly anticonvulsant drugs.

Selected Studies

Many studies highlight the benefit of supplementation with L-carnitine and its affiliated compounds, such as propionyl-L-carnitine, for the treatment of angina and other cardiovascular disorders. Propionyl-L-carnitine is taken up into the heart muscle cells more readily than other forms of carnitine. However, we will focus on L-carnitine, the most widely available and least expensive of this family of supplements.

L-carnitine supplementation improves overall oxygen utilization by the heart cells. Having enough L-carnitine available to metabolize fatty acids efficiently lets the heart do more with less oxygen. Without enough, an accumulation of toxic free fatty acid metabolites inside the cells can develop even before symptoms of angina are felt. The mitochondria become paralyzed. ATP levels crash. Energy reserves become depleted.

Usually, an increase in physical output triggers angina symptoms. So a great way to gauge the impact of L-carnitine in angina patients is to use exercise studies. In one study, the therapeutic effect was evaluated on two hundred patients over a six-month period. The patients, ranging from forty to sixty-five, all had pronounced exercise-induced angina. In the experiment they all received their regular drug regimen, but some were given a daily dose of 2 grams of L-carnitine. When the researchers compared the two groups at the end of the study, they found the supplemented patients had a significant reduction in EKG evidence of ischemia and ventricular ectopic contractions (skipped heartbeats) along with an increased tolerance to exercise. The results confirmed improved cardiac performance. In addition, the supplemented patients reported improved quality of life.

The potential of intravenous L-carnitine in emergency cardiology to protect heart attack survivors has emerged in recent years thanks to an ongoing Italian multicenter study. The results released so far indicate that supplementation in the early stages of a heart attack limits the damage of the infarct, reduces arrhythmia, and protects against chamber enlargement that may lead to aneurysm formation.

Perhaps the most promising potential of L-carnitine in cardiovascular conditions has been its ability, along with CoQ10 and D-ribose, to reduce the high death rate among end-stage heart failure patients. These individuals often have had several heart attacks, resulting in so much scar tissue that little remains of healthy, functioning heart muscle tissue. Some patients may have cardiomyopathy as well—the heart is stretched out, dilated, and enlarged, often the result of longstanding high blood pressure. Other cases may result from valvular problems, viruses that have attacked the heart muscle, toxic metal overload, or generalized atherosclerosis. All too often, heart failure and cardiomyopathy are *idiopathic*, meaning we really don't know the causes.

L-carnitine helps rescue such compromised hearts through its fatty acid transportation role. Three recent studies have shown that damaged heart tissue has trouble holding onto its L-carnitine, creating a deficiency that directly impacts heart function. The studies showed that supplementation compensates for this undesirable situation and improves blood pressure, cholesterol levels, rhythm disorders, and signs and symptoms of heart failure. In one study among 160 patients, researchers found that the incidence of death was 1.2 percent for L-carnitine–supplemented patients compared to 12.5 percent for the nonsupplemented group!

Patients with heart failure may have energy levels 30 percent lower than normal. In this condition, oxygenated blood doesn't flow effectively to peripheral muscles, leaving an energy shortfall in the extremities that compounds fatigue and the inability to perform even the simplest of life's daily activities. The whole body suffers. L-carnitine, as well as CoQ10 and D-ribose, contribute to energy improvement not just in the heart muscle but systemically as well, including working skeletal muscle. All the mitochondria in the body benefit.

L-carnitine lowers triglycerides and in some patients the Lp(a) level. It helps maintain a healthy level of hemoglobin in patients with kidney disease. Just as with CoQ10, L-carnitine supplementation doesn't produce side effects.

Our Recommendations

For general prevention, particularly for vegetarians, we suggest 250 to 750 mg daily of L-carnitine. Our heart disease patients take 1 to 2 grams once or twice a day. It is best taken on an empty stomach. If this produces gastrointestinal distress, take it with food. There's no significant advantage in taking more than 2 grams at any one time because saturation of intestinal mucosa occurs at this dosage level.

The two most common preparations you'll find in a health food store are the fumarates and the tartrates. We prefer L-carnitine fumarate over L-carnitine tartrate because we have found it to be more efficient, especially for patients with oxygen-starved hearts.

SigmaTau U.S., an offshoot of an Italian pharmaceutical company specializing in carnitine research, has led the development of promising combinations of L-carnitine and different amino acids such as L-arginine, glycine, and lysine. These new forms—called AminoCarnitines—may have increased therapy relevance. For example, L-carnitine arginate is a combination of L-carnitine and the amino acid L-arginine. L-arginine stimulates nitric oxide production, as we have seen, resulting in improved arterial dilation. The combination produces both dilation and energy effects attractive for individuals with CVD and male sexual dysfunction. For more information on this new technology, visit the SigmaTau Web site: www.sigmatau.com.

D-ribose

D-ribose is the new kid on the heart supplement block. As a building block of ATP, it rapidly restores depleted energy in sick hearts.

You probably haven't heard about D-ribose. But you will. It's that good. Every cell in the human body makes some of this simple sugar molecule, but only slowly and to varying degrees, depending on the tissue. The liver, adrenal glands, and fat tissue produce the most—enough to serve their purpose of making compounds involved in the production of hormones and fatty acids. But tissue elsewhere has little.

Red meat, particularly veal, contains the highest dietary concentration of D-ribose, but not significant enough to provide any meaningful nutritional support, especially to unwell individuals. Heart, skeletal muscle, brain, and nerve tissue can only make enough D-ribose to manage their day-to-day needs when their cells are not stressed. Unfortunately, these cells lack the metabolic machinery to make D-ribose quickly when they come under metabolic stress such as blood and oxygen deprivation (ischemia). When oxygen or blood flow deficits are chronic, as in heart disease, tissues can never make enough D-ribose. Cellular energy levels become depleted. D-ribose is the only compound used by the human body to replenish the diminished ATP energy stores.

The Doctor as Guinea Pig

When Dr. Roberts heard about D-ribose, a lightbulb immediately went on in his head. For some time, he had been using L-carnitine and CoQ10 in his medical practice to boost energy metabolism in sick hearts, but neither L-carnitine nor CoQ10 can rebuild the metabolic energy pool once it has been depleted by heart disease. He wondered if D-ribose could be the missing link.

Before trying it on patients, he decided to try it first on himself. As a marathon runner, he knows the importance of energy recovery. It is the impaired recovery of the muscle ATP pool that causes the pain, soreness, stiffness, and fatigue that follow long-distance training runs. He found that taking D-ribose before and after a run eliminated these problems. The usual muscle pain and soreness that persist for a day or two, or even three, were gone. He was no longer fatigued in the days after a hard workout. He was convinced!

In his cardiology practice, he offers patients an enhanced external counterpulsation (EECP) program, a noninvasive method that restores the flow of oxygenated blood in patients with recurrent or inoperable coronary artery disease (more about this method in chapter 12). Before D-ribose, most of the patients on EECP experienced *good* improvement. After adding D-ribose, improvement made a quantum leap to *great*. In hard-core cases like these, supplying oxygen alone to the chronically flow-deprived heart cells was not enough. Yes, the cells were deficient in CoQ10 and L-carnitine, but above all they lacked the precursors of ATP.

He began to put patients with angina and heart failure on D-ribose. They also improved. Time after time, Dr. Roberts found remarkable improvement in cardiac function measurements, exercise tolerance, quality of life, and recovery from fatigue. He was hooked and soon was lecturing about D-ribose at medical meetings.

The ABCs of D-ribose

Ischemia may cause the heart to lose up to 50 percent of its ATP pool. Even if blood flow and oxygen are restored to normal levels, it may take up to ten days for an otherwise healthy animal heart to rebuild cellular energy and normalize diastolic cardiac function. In studies, when oxygen-starved animals receive D-ribose, energy recovery and diastolic function return to normal in an average of two days. When patients with CAD are treated with D-ribose, symptoms and treadmill time improve significantly within one week.

Several factors determine who should take D-ribose supplements and when they should be taken. Age is one consideration. We believe 20 to 25 percent of people over forty-five, men and women alike, show early signs of diastolic cardiac dysfunction (stiff heart) and are at risk of contracting heart failure later in life. This is especially true in people with high blood pressure, people taking statin drugs, and in women with severe mitral valve prolapse. For these people, D-ribose supplementation increases the cardiac energy reserve and helps the heart restore normal diastolic cardiac function.

We also know that the health of our mitochondria suffers as we age. As a result, even minor metabolic stress can have a dramatic effect on cellular energy stores in an aging population.

Patients with heart disease on drugs intended to increase the contractile strength of their heart are also good candidates for D-ribose. These drugs, known as inotropic agents, make the heart beat harder. This places considerable strain on the heart's ability to supply enough energy to support the extra metabolic stress. Long-term treatment with these agents drains the energy reserve, essentially running the heart out of energy. Patients with heart failure, chronic coronary artery disease, or cardiomyopathy should take D-ribose to offset the energy-draining effects of inotropic drugs such as Digoxin. Research shows that supplementation reduces the energy drain without any negative impact on the activity of the drug.

Patients with coronary artery disease and persistent symptoms remain in a chronic state of energy depletion, constantly fatigued, weak, and with their heart function progressively worsening. These patients will almost certainly advance into congestive heart failure without improvement of the energy state of their heart. Restoration of their energy pool can only be accomplished through the pathway of energy metabolism regulated by the availability of D-ribose.

We cannot overstate the effect of D-ribose supplementation on maintaining energy levels. Any tissue that relies heavily on aerobic energy metabolism, such as the heart and muscles, will be severely affected by any amount of oxygen deprivation. The problem is ATP drain. The solution is to give it back!

Fibromyalgia patients are chronically fatigued and subject to muscle pain, soreness, and stiffness that can be associated with depleted cellular energy reserves. We are learning that patients with fibromyalgia and chronic fatigue syndrome have faulty ATP metabolism, so it makes perfect sense to use D-ribose to help them.

Unlike many other nutrients, we can't really talk about a formal D-ribose deficiency in tissue. Deficiencies refer to tissue concentrations of nutrients that fall to below-normal levels. D-ribose is not stored in cells in its free form; thus, there is no "normal" level of D-ribose in tissue. Instead, cells are faced with the task of making D-ribose in response to a specific metabolic demand. And this is where they get into trouble, because making D-ribose is a slow and time-consuming process in virtually all cells.

"You Fixed Louis"

Louis came to Dr. Sinatra's office suffering from severe coronary artery disease. Although previously treated with a stent placed in his left anterior descending artery, he still had severe blockage in an important arterial branch called the diagonal. The branch would have been difficult to dilate with a stent and unreasonable to bypass with surgery.

Louis had stubborn angina because of this unresolved situation. He experienced chest pain with normal activity, such as walking across a room, or from just mild emotional stress. He had visited several cardiologists for his heart problem. They gave him a number of standard heart drugs, but his situation persisted, and he decided to see Dr. Sinatra for a fresh opinion.

Testing showed that Louis had high levels of uric acid in his blood, indicating faulty ATP metabolism. He had already been taking low doses of L-carnitine and CoQ10. He needed higher doses, and he needed D-ribose to build his ATP pool. In just a few days, Louis showed such remarkable improvement that his son-in-law called and reported, "You fixed Louis!"

The Rise of D-ribose

Until 1944, D-ribose was thought to be primarily a structural component of DNA and RNA with little physiological significance. But a series of studies, culminating in 1957, revealed that this sugar molecule played an intermediate role in an important metabolic reaction called the *pentose phosphate pathway*. This reaction is central to energy synthesis, the production of genetic material, and for providing substances used by certain tissues to make fatty acids and hormones.

The D-ribose connection to cardiac function was made by the physiologist Heinz-Gerd Zimmer at the University of Munich. In 1973, he reported that energy-starved hearts could recover faster if D-ribose was given prior to, or immediately following, ischemia (oxygen deprivation). Five years later, he reported the same effect in skeletal muscle and also showed for the first time that the energy-draining effects of drugs that make the heart beat more strongly (inotropic agents) could be lessened if

D-ribose was given along with the drug. Zimmer and his research colleagues later proved that D-ribose was the limiting element in energy recovery in ischemic tissue and that energy synthesis could not occur without it.

Zimmer's research sparked a flurry of research on humans, rats, rabbits, guinea pigs, dogs, and even turkeys, all with similar results. D-ribose administration significantly improved energy recovery in ischemic, hypoxic, or cardiomyopathic hearts and skeletal muscle, and it improved functional performance of the tissue. In addition, studies with several common heart drugs—those used even today—showed that D-ribose administration did not negatively affect (and in many cases helped) the action of the drug on the heart.

The most significant findings of the studies underscored the dramatic effect that D-ribose administration played in both energy restoration and the return of normal diastolic cardiac function. A clinical study from Zimmer's group in Munich in 1992 showed that D-ribose administration to patients with severe, stable coronary artery disease increased exercise tolerance and delayed the onset of moderate angina. Since this groundbreaking study in coronary artery disease, the benefits of D-ribose have been reported for cardiac surgery recovery, heart failure and neuromuscular disease treatment, restoration of energy to stressed skeletal muscle, and control of free radical formation in oxygen-deprived tissue.

Several notable papers were published in 2003. One study showed that D-ribose improved diastolic functional performance of the heart, increased exercise tolerance, and significantly improved the quality of life of patients. Researchers have even extended their sights to healthy hearts and bodies and documented benefit from D-ribose supplements to improve athletic performance.

Research continues here and abroad. Yet, despite the powerful scientific evidence, very few U.S. physicians have even heard of D-ribose outside of their first-year medical school biochemistry class, and fewer still recommend it to patients. We lucky ones who are familiar with it have the wonderful gratification of seeing it help our patients on a regular basis.

Our Recommendations

Supplemental D-ribose absorbs easily and quickly through the gut and into the bloodstream. About 97 percent gets through.

How much D-ribose do you need? That question can only be answered with another question, "What do you want it to do for you?"

Studies have shown that *any* amount of D-ribose you give to energy-starved cells gives them an energy boost. At the University of Missouri, researcher Ronald Terjung has shown that even very small doses (the equivalent of about 500 mg) of D-ribose increase energy salvage in muscles by more than 100 percent. Larger doses increase the production of energy compounds by 340 to 430 percent, depending on the type of muscle tested, and improve the salvage of energy compounds by up to 650 percent. Most amazing is that when muscles are supplemented with D-ribose, they continue to add to their energy stores even while they actively work! Until this study was reported, it was thought that muscle energy stores were only refilled in muscles at rest.

An adequate dose of D-ribose usually results in symptom improvement very quickly—sometimes within a few days. If the initial response is poor, the dose should be increased until the patient feels relief. Logically, the sickest patients stand to gain the most.

Patients with arterial and heart disease who chronically choke off oxygen delivery to their tissues need to take a higher dosage simply to allow enough of it to work its way through the clogged vessels into the energy-parched portions of the heart. We start those patients at higher dosages and monitor their progress. With progress, the dosage can be reduced to the lowest possible point at which good energy and quality of life are maintained.

Those patients must take D-ribose every day. Missing even one or two days will negatively impact cellular energy, which will show up as weakness and fatigue.

D-ribose comes in various formulations: powders, beverages, tablets, energy bars, and other forms. We don't know the optimal level for every patient or every pathological condition, but we can make some recommendations as dosage starting points:

- 5 grams (if using a powder, two teaspoons) daily for cardiovascular prevention, for athletes on maintenance, and for healthy people doing strenuous activity

- 10 to 15 grams daily for most patients with heart failure, other forms of ischemic cardiovascular disease, peripheral vascular disease, individuals recovering from heart surgery or heart attack, for treatment of stable angina, and for athletes working out in chronic bouts of high-intensity exercise

- 15 to 30 grams daily for patients with advanced heart failure, dilated cardiomyopathy, or frequent angina, individuals awaiting heart transplant, and people with fibromyalgia or neuromuscular disease

Start at the upper level of each range for patients with heart or peripheral vascular disease. We recommend that daily doses up to 10 grams be taken as two 5 gram doses with morning and evening meals or just before and just after exercise or activity. Larger doses (15 grams per day or more) should be taken in three or sometimes even four smaller doses of about 5 grams each. Daily doses in excess of 30 grams are seldom needed. Most heart patients will stabilize at about 10 grams per day.

Once a patient responds with a reduction in symptoms, the dosage may be gradually reduced until a maintenance level is reached. Sometimes patients well maintained at a certain dose may require an increase due to changes in their activity level or changes in their cardiac drug therapy, such as the addition or deletion of beta blockers or calcium channel blockers. It cannot be overemphasized that patients must continue on D-ribose therapy, or relapses will almost certainly occur. D-ribose is quickly absorbed and leaves the blood rapidly. Therefore, assessing blood levels of D-ribose is not helpful in addition to being very costly.

Precautions

The toxicology and safety of D-ribose have been exhaustively studied. The supplement is 100 percent safe when taken as directed. Thousands of patients have taken D-ribose at dosages up to 60 grams per day with minimal side effects. However, even though there are no known contraindications of D-ribose therapy, we recommend that pregnant women, nursing mothers, and very young children refrain from taking D-ribose simply because there is not enough research on its use in these populations.

D-ribose can actually lower blood glucose levels; therefore, insulin-dependent diabetics should check with their physicians before starting on the supplement. Carefully monitor the blood glucose level so as not to accidentally overdose on insulin. We have had no problems recommending D-ribose to insulin-dependent diabetics when the supplement is taken with orange juice.

Reported side effects are minimal and infrequent. Patients may experience light-headedness if they take a large dosage (10 grams or more) on a completely empty stomach. Take D-ribose with meals, or at least mixed into juice, milk, or fruit, to offset the blood glucose–lowering effect.

There are no known adverse drug or nutritional interactions associated with D-ribose use.

Chapter 8

Detox

Beginning in the 1930s, research chemists became interested in the ability of certain amino acids to form stable bonds with metals. New compounds were developed, first for industrial use and then for medical use. One of them was a synthetic compound called EDTA (ethylenediaminetetraacetic acid), which proved effective as an antidote to heavy metal toxicity such as lead poisoning. When infused into the bloodstream, this substance chelated—that is, grabbed onto minute particles of lead and escorted them out of the body through the urine.

EDTA treatment gained importance during the 1950s for lead poisoning among workers in battery factories and sailors in the U.S. Navy who painted ships with lead-based paint. The effectiveness and safety of the method prompted the FDA to approve of EDTA chelation for lead poisoning.

Doctors soon began reporting improvement in the circulatory status of EDTA-treated patients with chronic lead poisoning who also had arterial plaque deposits. The reports spawned an interest in chelation therapy among many physicians to help patients with CVD.

Today, more than a thousand doctors worldwide use chelation therapy for a variety of CVD-related conditions. The method not only clears lead from the system but also excess iron, cadmium, aluminum, and other harmful metals that can poison enzyme systems in the body.

Chelation involves a painless intravenous procedure that drips EDTA into the circulation during a series of twenty to forty office treatments. The IV also contains magnesium, vitamin C, and B vitamins. Patients sit comfortably during these sessions, reading or watching TV.

Proponents believe that removal of toxic metals, among other benefits, restores the ability of endothelial cells to produce the nitric oxide necessary for healthy arterial dilation and to fend off free radical activity. Toxic metals irreversibly damage enzyme systems and are associated with an increased risk of high blood pressure and plaque formation. Supporters feel that metal overload plays a key role in CVD, malignancy, and many other age-related chronic diseases.

For more than forty years, physicians have repeatedly reported in medical journals on the benefits of chelation therapy, including a significant improvement in blood flow and symptoms for patients with atherosclerosis, angina, circulatory disorders, hypertension, and diabetes. Chelating doctors include dietary changes—such as avoiding highly refined and processed foods—and nutritional supplementation in their treatment.

Carefully controlled scientific studies, however, have been lacking, and although many doctors use chelation for toxic metal removal in CVD patients, the application per se for CVD has not been officially sanctioned. It is, in fact, opposed by medical organizations such as the American Heart Association. Medical insurers, including Medicare, will not cover the procedure. Practitioners who use chelation believe this resistance arises from fear of competition within the medical establishment, and specifically that chelation threatens the economics of entrenched therapies, such as pharmaceuticals and surgery.

In an attempt to clear up the controversy, the National Heart, Lung, and Blood Institute of the National Institutes of Health has launched the first large-scale study of EDTA chelation therapy for patients with coronary artery disease. More than a hundred centers, clinics, and doctors' offices are participating in this five-year placebo-controlled double-blind study that began in 2003.

We know that chelation works with kidney disease, in which toxic metals such as lead and cadmium damage the enzymes in the kidneys, leading slowly to kidney failure. Patients with damaged kidneys improve or stabilize, as shown in randomized controlled studies. The assumption is that chelation removes the offending metals. We feel the same thing happens with compromised arteries to the heart, in which the metals undermine arterial dilation and antioxidant enzyme systems. They also poison the enzymes involved in generating energy. CoQ10, L-carnitine, and D-ribose can't work well if the enzymes that process them are poisoned.

From Dr. Roberts's Chelation Files

I have seen patients with otherwise inoperable disease benefit greatly from IV chelation therapy that I performed as a last-ditch effort. These were situations in which nothing else worked and I was totally stuck.

My first chelation case was about ten years ago, and the experience sold me on the technique. Mary, a sixty-five-year-old patient, had had bypass surgery following a heart attack. The surgery failed. Her symptoms returned. She had constant angina. We tried angioplasty. It failed as well. The arteries narrowed again.

Today, I could try quite a few different options with her, but with my knowledge at that time I felt I had reached a dead end. She was on maximum medication and still having pain. I suggested she consider a heart transplant. She was put on a waiting list, but the medical team didn't think they would be able to get to her for six months.

Mary had heard about chelation and asked if I could give it to her. I told her I didn't know how to do it and that it was controversial. She said she still wanted to try and felt it could help her, but I would be the only one who she would let do it. I was very concerned about her not lasting to the date of the transplant, so I took a course in chelation therapy. I obtained the necessary materials to perform the treatment.

The treatment stabilized her condition for the necessary six months, long enough for Mary to get her transplant. I was surprised that the therapy worked so well when all my conventional methods had not.

As Mary sat in the office getting her series of treatments, some other patients noticed what was happening. Several approached me and said they had been getting chelation elsewhere and were doing well on it. Because of the controversial nature of chelation therapy, they didn't want to tell me about it—that is, until they saw Mary receiving the therapy in my office.

Over time, I learned that a number of my patients had been receiving chelation therapy from another doctor. These were individuals who I had strongly urged to have open heart surgery because I felt surgery was the only option to keep them alive.

As the months went on and I noticed that these patients were looking pretty good, I wanted to know what was going on. Sheepishly, they admitted getting chelation from a different physician and feeling better as a result. They hadn't told me because they thought I would throw them out of my practice. At that time, most cardiologists would not accept chelating patients.

The improvements I saw with Mary and now with other patients getting chelation without my knowledge motivated me to learn more about this technique. I started doing more and more chelation treatments and indeed saw my patients improve. The benefits of IV chelation became obvious to me. Many of my patients made complete turnarounds with IV chelation added to their therapy.

Take Dave, for instance, who I first saw in 1997 when he was fifty-five. He had undergone two rounds of angioplasty and had two stents placed in another artery. Abdominal aortic and popliteal artery (the artery behind the knee) aneurysms had been repaired. Blood flow to his lower extremities was poor, causing leg cramping when walking. On top of all this, chest pain remained an issue. An angiogram revealed 50 percent narrowings in all three of his coronary vessels.

Dave came to me for a second opinion. He was taking a number of drugs, including a statin cholesterol-lowering agent. These were continued. But a program of antioxidants, minerals, and L-carnitine were added along with weekly IV chelation.

Dave's symptoms improved. Then they resolved. His noninvasive vascular studies haven't changed in eight years nor has he required a cardiovascular-related hospital admission or any further vascular surgery. He was troubled by shortness of breath in mid-2005 (which turned out to be due to asthma), and a stress test returned mildly abnormal. Fearing that Dave's coronary disease had progressed, I repeated his coronary angiogram. The blood pressure within the heart was normal and his arteries looked better than in 1997. The worst narrowing was only 40 percent. This man had undergone six previous vascular procedures, but with chelation his disease state was arrested. Blood flow improved and remained improved over eight years.

Bill, another patient, had a heart attack in 1986 followed by bypass surgery. He was seventy-five. Afterward, he learned all he could about nutritional medicine and began a supplement program along with IV chelation.

In 2000, he developed chest pain. It turned out he was going through a stressful period in his life and had inadvertently gone off several of his medications. I repeated his coronary angiogram and saw three pristine grafts. Normally, one in three vein grafts close within one year and half close within seven years. But all three of Bill's grafts looked great at fourteen years.

My patient June required single-vessel stent placement in 1997, when she was seventy. The stent failed, and two years later she underwent multivessel bypass surgery, complicated by a heart attack. Her arteries were very small, and she was told that further intervention would not be possible. She also had a 3.4 cm abdominal aortic aneurysm (an abnormal blood-filled dilation of an artery caused by disease of the vessel wall). A normal diameter is less than 2 to 2.5 cm. We operate at 5 to 6 cm or if the aneurysm expands rapidly.

Angina recurred in mid-1999. That's when June came in for a second opinion. I added my basic nutritional program along with chelation therapy.

Her angina improved. A repeat ultrasound in 2002 showed her aneurysm had decreased to 2.4 cm. This allowed us to treat June with enhanced external counterpulsation, the technique I use to restore oxygenated blood flow in patients with continuing or inoperable coronary artery disease.

Through the spring of 2005, June has logged a hundred chelation treatments. She hasn't required hospitalization. Her aorta remains at 2.4 cm. The radiologists no longer describe it as an aneurysm but as a borderline enlarged aorta. EDTA chelation therapy helped an inoperable coronary patient improve her quality of life.

No-Hassle Oral Chelation

There are, however, a few downsides to IV chelation. First, patients spend three hours at a time sitting in the doctor's office while an IV drips EDTA into their veins. They often require thirty or more such treatments, enough to clear their toxic metal burden. Second, medical insurers won't cover it. Nor will Medicare. Another problem is that patients sometimes develop irritated veins from the repeated procedure. So it is unsatisfactory for quite a few people.

Recently, however, a significant oral chelation formula has been developed that works well: DetoxMaxPlus. We described it at length in chapter 6, under the section on phosphatidylcholine.

DetoxMaxPlus contains EDTA, which binds and removes toxic

metals, along with the arterial nourishing effects of phosphatidylcholine in a combined formula. This is chelation in a more convenient and less expensive form.

Whatever the technique—oral or IV—to rid the body of toxic minerals, this is a needed treatment in medicine. It is critical to detoxify patients. If we can reduce high blood pressure by taking away heavy metals, this is better than prescribing a drug. The effect will last longer. Once you start on a drug for blood pressure, doctors will always increase the dosage. And then you will get another prescription.

Heavy metals appear to play a role in high cholesterol as well. They poison the enzymes of reverse cholesterol transport.

From Dr. Roberts's Oral Chelation Files

Kathy was one of my first DetoxMaxPlus patients. She was seventy-six when I first saw her, with multiple risk factors including high blood pressure.

Previously, she had sustained a minor heart attack. Her angiogram showed severe disease in all three coronary arteries. Bypass surgery was recommended, but Kathy wanted to explore other approaches first. Another physician put her on a program that included drug therapy, an extensive nutritional regimen, and IV chelation.

The program kept Kathy out of the hospital but didn't resolve her symptoms. She was still doing poorly after eleven chelation treatments and had shortness of breath with mild activity. Her stress test was abnormal at a low exercise level.

I felt she needed open heart surgery, and I pushed for it as her best option. I was worried about her. She refused and said matter-of-factly, "I hear you have something better."

I put her on DetoxMaxPlus. Four months later, I saw her again. Kathy's energy level was better. Her blood pressure was lower, and she told me she was mowing her backyard with a push lawn mower. Her symptoms essentially disappeared in four months. She has kept up with this program and remains asymptomatic more than two years later. She hasn't set foot in a hospital.

Another very positive case involved Hazel, a seventy-four-year-old hypertensive patient with multiple risk factors. Despite comprehensive medication, she had a cholesterol reading of 368 and progressive claudication (walking-related leg pain due to lower extremity vascular disease). Her symptoms and ultrasound test scores were gradually deteriorating.

She, too, was another candidate for surgery, but again I decided to try a therapy program built around DetoxMaxPlus. Like Kathy, Hazel's symptoms improved quickly. She felt better in six weeks. Her medical workups showed major improvement, foremost among them a standard test to determine the adequacy of blood flow to the legs. We do this test by looking at the ratio of arm and ankle blood pressure readings. If the leg blood flow is much lower than the flow to the arm, we know there's a problem. Initially, Hazel registered only 30 percent in her leg, compared to her arm flow. Now she is up to 50 percent of normal and is walking as far as she wants without discomfort. She shops and goes about her business normally. Her cholesterol fell. Her atherosclerosis is essentially being reversed.

I have had quite a few dramatic outcomes among the more than two hundred or so patients for whom I have prescribed DetoxMaxPlus. I have found that (1) it does remove heavy metals, and (2) it does improve symptoms and blood flow.

Carotid ultrasounds are healthier. Each patient with angina has less chest pain. There are almost across-the-board improvements. Keep in mind, however, that I use this with the rest of my program and never alone. I continue to use IV chelation but am somewhat frustrated by the cost and the time factor. Now I am delighted to have an oral supplement that people can take at home.

Our Recommendations

We regard DetoxMaxPlus as a terrific option for patients with inoperable heart disease where nothing else works and basically for anyone with symptomatic CVD and plaque.

DetoxMaxPlus is only available through doctors at this time through the manufacturer (BioImmune, Scottsdale, Arizona, 888-663-8844). You'll need to work with your physician.

Another newly available oral chelation product similar to DetoxMax Plus is called Pegaflo Detox. It can be obtained for patients by doctors through BioMolecular Sciences in Marina del Rey, California (800-260-3587 or www.genomicwhey.com).

The Lowdown on Lead

Science tells us that lead is poisoning the brains of our children, driving up our blood pressure, and damaging our kidneys. Yet the way most physicians test for lead is ineffective. The standard procedure measures blood lead levels, which invariably come back in the "safe" range. Patients are then told that lead is not a problem.

The problem with lead lies elsewhere. It is not stored in the blood. It accumulates within cells, tightly bound to structural proteins. Thus, blood lead levels do not reflect the body burden of lead in adults.

If you have CVD, and especially high blood pressure or kidney disease, consider consulting with a physician trained in heavy metal toxicology who can accurately test for—and remove—lead and other harmful metals. You can find a directory of physicians through the American College for Advancement in Medicine (call 800-532-3688 or visit the organization's Web site at www.acam.org) or the International College of Integrative Medicine (call 866-464-5226 or visit www.icimed.com).

Sweat the Small (Metal) Stuff—Out

By raising your body's temperature, the sauna is a perfect way to open your pores and promote the departure of toxic substances from the body. Heat forces toxic materials out of cells, so they can be excreted through the sweat glands. Saunas also enhance microcirculation, moving more oxygen to injured tissues, and can help encourage a lessening of inflammation.

Sweating out mercury, for instance, has a long history. This technique was employed in Spain in the 1950s and 1960s. Miners who showed mental confusion and tremors, both clinical signs of mercury toxicity, were placed in hot environments and forced to sweat to get rid of the mercury.

A conventional sauna may be stressful for patients with advanced heart disease, but far infrared sauna (FIR), which provides the benefits of sauna at a lower temperature, is typically well tolerated. Studies have shown beneficial effects of FIR on endothelial function, heart rate variability and rhythm, ejection fraction, and symptomatic status in patients with heart failure. An excellent article on FIR, including how to build one for under $100 in your own home, appeared in the November 2002 issue of *Townsend Let-*

ter for Doctors and Patients (call the publication for a reprint at 360-385-6021 or download the article from the Internet at the Find Articles Web site: www.findarticles.com/p/articles/mi_m0ISW/is_2002_Nov/ai_93736414).

Use heat therapies with caution, and consume plenty of fluids to keep your body well hydrated during the process.

Chapter 9

The Anti-Inflammatory Diet

Let thy food be thy medicine and
thy medicine be thy food.

—HIPPOCRATES

There are so many different ways to eat. So many different diets. How can you not be confused?

In New Cardiology, we feel you need to eat an artery-friendly, anti-inflammatory diet—an eating plan that protects you from the silent and destructive inflammation that leads to dangerous plaque formation. For sure, it is way too easy to eat the bad stuff.

Like most cardiologists, we used to recommend that patients follow the American Heart Association guidelines, a diet low in fat and high in energy-releasing carbohydrates. The guidelines made sense to those of us in the medical establishment who believed that less fat in the diet would mean less fat in the bloodstream. We figured that carbohydrates, such as bread, pasta, and rice, would be beneficial or at the very least harmless. Unfortunately, it didn't work out quite the way we thought.

We later learned that replacing fat calories with typical carbohydrates actually *promotes* CVD because it stimulates the pancreas to produce more insulin. Insulin is an essential hormone that enables the body to absorb the breakdown products of carbohydrates and carry these substances as glucose—another name for blood sugar—into the cells to generate energy. Excessive quantities of carbohydrates, a result of high-carb, low-fat diets, requires more insulin to process the carbohydrates.

Too much insulin signals the body to store the overload of carbohydrates as fat. The more carbs you eat and the less active you are, the more the carbs turn into fat. That means more weight. The sad consequence of cozying up to carbs and becoming increasingly sedentary is that Americans have gotten fatter—there has been a 32 percent weight increase in the last ten years, and nearly two-thirds of the population is now considered overweight. The realization of what carbs hath wrought has inspired a seemingly endless production of low-carb diet books and revitalized the life of the high-protein classic, the Atkins diet.

We use the term *glycemic index* to characterize carbohydrate foods by the relative speed with which they are broken down into glucose for entry into the bloodstream and delivery to cells. Refer to the glycemic food index in appendix B. The rate of conversion determines the amount of insulin secreted by the pancreas to regulate carbohydrate metabolism. Foods with a high glycemic index—that is, more carbohydrate content per serving—require more insulin to be broken down. These foods include breads, potatoes, pastas, pastries, rice, and anything with high concentrations of sugar. We also use the term *refined carbohydrates*, meaning highly processed foods loaded with sugar. They give you that temporary sugar high, a spike in blood sugar, often followed by an energy crash when insulin rushes in to normalize the level. Candies, pies, pastries, and alcohol are particularly quick to enter into the system bulging with cargoes of sugar.

The rise in insulin triggers carbohydrate cravings. And when more carbs and sweets are eaten, this vicious cycle starts all over again. The food-addicted individual develops a need for continual quick fixes. The consequence is excessively high blood sugar and insulin production and an energy roller-coaster.

If this high tide of insulin becomes the digestive norm in your system, the insulin receptor sites on the membranes of cells, through which glucose passes, become damaged. The cells start to lose their ability to recognize insulin, leaving it to circulate and build up in the bloodstream. We call this situation insulin resistance and recognize it as a forerunner to type 2 diabetes and obesity.

In chapter 3, we introduced the damaging and inflammatory effects of this high blood sugar and insulin scenario. It's an overlooked yet very serious risk factor for developing unhealthy arteries and thick blood. Not just heart health is at stake but brain function as well.

It is vitally important that you regulate your insulin levels, reduce your glycemic load, and eliminate as many simple sugars as you can.

Introducing the PAM Diet

After all the technology we've developed in the last century to mass produce foods that are quick and easy, health professionals and health-conscious laypeople alike have come to recognize the danger that lurks beneath the convenience and slick packaging. We have learned to go back to the basics, to the wisdom of Hippocrates twenty-four hundred years ago, who observed that food was powerful medicine.

In our modern age, science has repeatedly validated the link between eating and health. Science is one thing. But we tend to learn more from our own experience—and mistakes. For many of us, it has taken making poor food choices that have led to less than good health to finally bring us back to the basics.

On the AHA diet, patients tended to develop insulin resistance. And despite our best intentions, even doctors like us gained weight and watched our cholesterol and triglyceride levels rise. It was alarming. There had to be better ways of eating that would offer better cardioprotective benefits.

The research led directly to two parts of the world: Asia and the Mediterranean regions of Italy, Greece, and Spain. Natives of these cultures experience a fraction of the cardiovascular illness seen in northern Europe and the United States. Of course, the most compelling statistics come from the years before these regions became Westernized and filled with that most dubious of American exports: fast-food restaurants. Thanks to the introduction of American junk food, younger generations abroad and those who have moved to the United States and don't follow their traditional diets see an incidence of cardiovascular disease catching up to our level.

The Mediterranean and Japanese people have some of the longest life expectancies in the world. When you examine their respective diets, the reason is apparent. Although the Mediterranean people do not eat much soy or seaweed, two very healthy components of Asian culture, and Asians don't eat olive oil, both diets have low levels of saturated and hydrogenated fats, higher levels of healthy fats, and an emphasis on fish and vegetables.

Combine the two and you have the best of both far-flung worlds: a potpourri of healthy, healing foods, including fresh vegetables, legumes, fruits, fish, garlic, nuts, olive oil, and soy products. We call it the Pan-Asian Mediterranean diet, or PAM for short, and recommend it to patients.

This type of diet is compatible with most of the principles underlying another popular diet plan that you probably have heard of: the Zone diet. Both are at odds with earlier diets that pushed high carbohydrates instead of highly processed and fatty foods. The PAM diet further recommends that even fewer of your calories come from lean protein and instead that more come from the healthy fats found in Asian and Mediterranean foods.

Both the Zone and PAM diets suggest you limit 40 percent of your caloric intake to carbs. The PAM plan emphasizes that they must be primarily low-glycemic carbs that don't stimulate your pancreas to flood the body with insulin. They also won't fan the fires of inflammation that consume your arteries. The idea is to eat so that your insulin engine is not running at full throttle.

The PAM approach to eating isn't a temporary diet plan. It is more a lifestyle specifically directed to the health of your arteries and heart, and generally to the smooth operation of your body as a whole. The central focus is making sure you combine the right balance of foods from the three food groups: carbohydrates, proteins, and fats. The suggested proportions are as follows:

- 40 percent low-density carbohydrates, such as most vegetables and low-glycemic fruits

- 25 to 30 percent organic protein, such as free-range meats, chicken, fish, tofu, or omega-3-fortified free-range eggs

- 30 to 35 percent monounsaturated fats, including but not limited to olive oil, nuts, tofu, fish, and avocado

The most important aspect of this plan is that you combine protein, carbohydrates, and fats according to this general equation in each meal to prevent an excessive insulin release. The plan thus rules out typical carbohydrate overloads like a big bowlful of sugared cereal with white bread toast and processed orange juice, or a serving of Italian bread followed by a plateful of pasta.

PAM: The Main Ingredients

1. Low-glycemic vegetables, grains, and fresh fruits. The best way to keep insulin and blood sugar levels low is to eat carbohydrates that rank low on the glycemic index. These foods usually contain more fiber (roughage). As it travels through the digestive tract, fiber cleanses the intestines, encourages regular bowel movements to keep your colon healthy, and gives you a feeling of fullness. Studies have shown that for every 10-gram increase of daily fiber, there is a stunning 29 percent reduction in the risk of heart disease. The best foods for lowering insulin are legumes (such as lentils and chickpeas) and broccoli.

2. High in antioxidants. Ample amounts of vegetables and fruits also deliver protective antioxidants and other micronutrients to the body. These naturally occurring compounds help combat free radical–induced diseases, including cataracts, cancer, CVD, and premature aging. Remember that LDL cholesterol isn't dangerous by itself. It's only when it becomes oxidized (through exposure to free radicals) that it becomes a danger to the arterial system. As we have seen in previous chapters, oxidized LDL molecules irritate the vessel walls, making them puffy and inflamed, and promote the development of fatty streaks and plaque. Even if your LDL level is high, antioxidants can help block this harmful process.

We have discussed antioxidant supplements. In food, the following fruits and vegetables pack the highest concentrations of antioxidants:

- Fruits: prunes (the most by far), raisins, blueberries, blackberries, strawberries, raspberries, plums, oranges, red grapes, and cherries

- Vegetables: kale, spinach, brussels sprouts, alfalfa sprouts, broccoli florets, beets, red bell peppers, onions, corn, and eggplant

Antioxidant compounds found in fruits and vegetables include flavonoids. They have impressive benefits for the whole body, particularly the cardiovascular system. Onions, for instance, are the best dietary source of quercetin, a flavonoid compound that helps block the oxidation of LDL. A Dutch study with men aged sixty-five to eighty-four found a reduced risk of heart attack and sudden death among those individuals who ate more onions.

If you like red wine, as many Mediterraneans do, you will be pleased to know about red wine polyphenols, compounds that change the properties of blood lipids to make LDL more resistant to oxidation. Moderate wine drinkers have a significantly lower mortality rate from coronary heart disease. Reservatrol, an antioxidant enzyme present in the lining of the grape, has been suggested as the antidote for keeping the incidence of French cardiovascular disease at a low level despite a typically fat-rich diet.

From the Asian drinking tradition we recommend green tea. In a coronary artery study of nearly five hundred Japanese men, those who drank at least one cup a day had a significantly lower risk of acute heart disease than their counterparts who preferred other beverages. The important benefit you receive from a soothing cup of green tea is its natural COX-2–inhibiting effect (COX-2 is short for cyclooxygenase-2, an enzyme involved in inflammatory activity). Garlic, ginger, turmeric, oregano, and onions also help block this enzyme.

3. High levels of healthy omega-3 fatty acids. The body cannot make essential fatty acids, so we must consume them as dietary fats (or oils) in the right balance. They allow for the storage of energy, the absorption of vital nutrients and vitamins, the production of numerous hormones, and the smooth function of the body.

Dietary fats come in two basic forms: saturated and unsaturated. Saturated fats are found in meat, poultry, and whole-milk dairy products. We tend to eat too many of them, creating an increased risk for cardiovascular disease. They are high in arachidonic acid, a fatty acid that triggers inflammation in the system and exerts toxic effects on the mitochondria, the energy-generating structures inside cells.

Saturated means the fat is solid at room temperature. Unsaturated fats are liquid, and they are found in two basic forms: monounsaturated (for example, olive oil) and polyunsaturated (for example, fish and vegetable oils). The polyunsaturates contain essential fatty acids, nutrients used by the body as raw materials to produce a huge array of subsidiary fatty substances that perform countless basic functions. Among other roles, they are fundamental building blocks of cellular membranes and regulatory compounds that enhance or suppress disease processes.

There are two major essential fatty acids in polyunsaturated fats: alpha-linolenic acid and linoleic acid. They, in turn, are classified into families according to their molecular structure. The families go by the names omega-3 and omega-6.

We should be eating a proper balance of these fatty acids. But we don't. In fact, we haven't been doing a good job at this for a hundred years or more, which may partly explain why we have so much heart disease and other chronic illnesses that were not common in earlier times. Over the years, we have been consuming huge amounts of foods that have much more omega-6 content. This imbalance is the result of a steep rise in the use of certain vegetable oils such as corn, safflower, and sunflower. These oils are high in omega-6 fatty acids compared to omega-3s. Corn oil, for instance, has a ratio of 60 to 1. Safflower has a ratio of 77 to 1. Contributing to the imbalance as well is a typically high intake of processed foods and margarine, which are loaded with omega-6s. According to an illuminating 1997 study from Japan, an unparalleled rise in heart disease, depression, allergies, and autoimmune conditions has taken place since Western-type food, high in omega-6s, has become popular.

Experts say that the overall ratio of omega-6s to omega-3s in today's Western diet ranges from 20 or 30 to 1 instead of an evolutionary ratio of 1 or 2 to 1. This dietary shift has created an alarming imbalance that researchers believe may contribute to inflammation, blood clot formation, and blood vessel constriction. A balanced ratio in the diet is essential for normal growth and development.

Because the typical American diet contains such an overkill of omega-6 and its major component of linoleic acid, supplementation of omega-6 is not usually needed. But omega-3 is a different story. More and more physicians are recommending omega-3 supplements to patients. We've been doing it for years in the form of fish oil, which is high in the beneficial eicosapentaenoic acid (EPA) and docosahexaenoic acid (DHA).

4. More fish, less beef and dairy. Besides their saturated fat content, meat and dairy are high in methionine, an amino acid precursor to homocysteine. Too much homocysteine is a major promoter of arterial damage. Moreover, the homogenization of milk creates very small compounds that get inside blood vessels, causing inflammation and injury to the vessel walls.

The Pan-Asian Mediterranean diet emphasizes fish for its lean, healthy protein and anti-inflammatory oils. Just by eating the equivalent of a fatty fish meal once a week, according to research at the University of Washington, you ingest enough good fatty acids to reduce your risk by half of developing an initial heart attack compared to individuals who have no dietary intake of EPA and DHA. The right kind of fish (see our recommendations and caveats at the end of the chapter) are rich in EPA and DHA.

Lean organic or free-range chicken breasts are okay as well. If your meats are marbled with fat, you get a whopping dose of saturated fat. Lean free-range top round steak has the lowest amount of saturated fat in the beef category.

5. High in olive oil. According to Greek mythology, the goddess Athena endowed the olive tree with great healing powers. Modern medical science is now showing that she really knew her stuff! So much in fact that in 2004 the Food and Drug Administration permitted food containing olive oil to carry labels saying it may reduce the risk of coronary heart disease. Although limited, the evidence suggests that eating about 2 tablespoons (23 grams) of olive oil daily may reduce the risk of coronary heart disease due to the monounsaturated fat content. So a change as simple as sautéing food at a low heat in olive oil instead of butter may be much better for your heart.

Oleuropein and hydroxytyrosol, two compounds found in olive oil, are potent scavengers of destructive free radicals and also help block LDL oxidation. What's more, 2½ tablespoons of extra-virgin olive oil a day has been found to lower blood pressure, so patients may be able to decrease their dosage of antihypertensive drugs. Just a slight reduction in saturated fat intake, along with the use of olive oil, may markedly drop the requirement for medication.

6. Low sodium. The program limits the amount of salt used to season meals. A diet high in sodium increases water retention. In turn, the added volume of fluid forces the heart to work harder to move blood through the body.

7. Nuts and seeds. These often forgotten foods are rich in good essential fatty acids, healthy protein, and fiber. They contain phytosterols, compounds that inhibit the body's ability to absorb dietary cholesterol.

8. Garlic. Smelly but oh so healthy. Behind the odor are powerful healing compounds with scientifically proven benefits for CVD. Allicin is one, a compound that helps raise HDL; lower LDL, homocysteine, and blood pressure; and decrease platelet stickiness.

9. Soy. Soy products tend to help lower LDL, promote HDL, and lower blood pressure.

10. Weight loss. Last but certainly not least, you will be happy to know that the fats found on the PAM program—from sources such as olive oil, cold-water fish, eggs, and nuts—are not only healthy but sustain energy levels longer and help satisfy appetite better than high-carbohydrate foods. Following the program's guidelines helps prevent the spikes and drops in blood sugar associated with consumption of refined carbohydrates. Stable blood sugar results in reduced cravings for sweets and little or no desire to binge eat. Together, these characteristics help promote weight loss.

Diets that claim to reduce weight and protect the heart abound. They include the famous Atkins diet and the South Beach diet. Each has some virtue and obviously works to reduce weight. However, there are concerns.

The Atkins diet, for example, is too high in saturated fat, which is a long-term risk factor for cancer and heart disease—the very problem it claims to treat. It lowers HDL cholesterol and raises CRP. Although newer versions of the diet claim to be lower in fat, they still do not place sufficient emphasis on vegetables. People still take in about 60 percent of their diet in the form of fat and are not consuming sufficient quantities of fiber, omega-3 fatty acids, vitamins, and other nutrients. This amount of fat carries the risk of poisoning the body with pesticides and insecticides that ultimately end up in fatty tissue high in the food chain.

The same limitation holds true for the South Beach diet. Indeed, all the low-carbohydrate diets, now the craze, place excessive emphasis on protein (which can put you at risk for some health problems, including kidney problems) and give the false impression that you will be healthy if you cut down on carbohydrates. Food stores now have lo-carb nutrition bars, incorrectly implying that they can replace nutritious meals.

Getting On the PAM Program

Now you know the nuts and bolts of the plan, or rather the nuts and seeds. Starting the PAM program is pretty simple if you just keep the basic formula in mind. There's no need to count calories, which most people won't do, anyway.

Remember to try to divide the food up for each meal as 25 to 30 percent of the calories from protein, a similar amount from healthy fats, and about half from slow-burning, low-glycemic carbohydrates that include whole grains, fresh fruits, and vegetables.

For the average person, this breaks down to several servings of protein per day, two tablespoons of olive oil (on salads and vegetables), and five to seven servings of fruits, vegetables, nuts, seeds, and grains.

You'll find a lot of variety within the equation so that you can turn this into a long-term plan. Your challenge, however, is to keep out certain detrimental foods as much as possible.

Try to avoid the following:

- Sugary condiments such as jams, jellies, and cranberry sauce
- Sugary drinks such as regular soda and fruit juice
- Foods containing the unhealthy trans fats (one of the "dirty dozen" risk factors) and saturated fats, such as whole milk, hard cheeses (with the exception of Parmesan), margarine, mayonnaise, flavored and sweetened whole yogurt, sour cream, bacon, low-fat cheeses, and luncheon meats
- High-sodium/high-preservative processed foods, such as any prepared foods (TV dinners, microwavable meals), and canned and/or boxed goods (check the labels for sodium content)

Vital Choice Alaskan Wild Salmon

We wanted to share one particularly healthy, delicious, and quick fish dish. Vital Choice, a company in Alaska, specializes in pristine wild salmon containing no mercury, heavy metal, pesticides, or PCBs. You can order from the Washington-based company's Web site at www.vitalchoice.com or by phone at (800) 608-4825. Products are shipped frozen.

Take the fish out of the freezer and immerse in cold water for twenty minutes to thaw. Chop up some garlic, parsley, and cilantro. Mix together and sprinkle onto a dinner plate.

After thawing, sauté the fish lightly in a frying pan with a couple of tablespoons of olive oil. You might want to choose a light olive oil that has a higher heat point, or organic coconut oil.

Sear the salmon for two minutes on each side. Flip the fish back and forth a few times, adding some pepper and garlic. Place the fish on the plate over the bed of garlic, parsley, and cilantro. Add two tablespoons of olive oil and freshly squeezed lemon juice. An accompanying salad makes a great combination.

Given the importance of fish oil, we think that eating healthy, migratory, and nonpolluted fish is a must for your diet. This is a great way to get it.

- Processed carbohydrate sources, such as refined cereals, cookies, chips, crackers, pasta, bread, and cake mixes made from white flour, instant mashed potatoes, gelatin, and pudding mixes

- All oils with the exception of walnut, almond, extra-virgin olive oil, and fish oils

- All sweeteners (including artificial sweeteners) with the exception of a dab of pure honey and the supplement stevia

As you discard the bad, you'll want to substitute with the good:

- If you feel a desire to drink milk, choose organic skim milk. Actually, there's not much need for milk because you get plenty of calcium from vegetables. A single serving of kale, for instance, contains as much calcium as a glass of milk.

- You can add low-fat organic yogurt, soy milk, organic fresh eggs, fat-free cottage cheese, and imported Parmesan cheese. After a few weeks, a small block of feta cheese or a package of soy cheese can be added.

- Look for fresh lemons, dark green lettuce, broccoli, spinach, blueberries, cantaloupe, tomatoes, cucumbers, onions, garlic, and celery. When in season, choose eggplant and red and green peppers.

- Choose skinless, boneless chicken breasts and turkey breasts. And try to buy free-range and antibiotic/hormone-free poultry.

- Fresh fish tastes best. Avoid farm-raised fish because they contain antibiotics (used to protect them from disease in overcrowded pens), as well as disturbing concentrations of pesticides and mercury. Stay away from the larger deep-sea fish such as swordfish, large tuna, and shark because of high levels of mercury and PCBs (polychlorinated biphenyls). If buying canned fish, avoid products packed with vegetable or cottonseed oil. Water or olive oil is preferable. Salmon, herring, halibut, lake trout, mackerel, sardines, and even anchovies are all high in omega-3s. As a bonus, fish is also a rich source of CoQ10.

- For flavor, use a selection of vinegars (red wine, balsamic), as well as fresh basil, oregano, bay leaf, marjoram, thyme, rosemary, and fennel. Asian seasonings include coriander seeds, cardamom pods, cumin, ground ginger, sesame seeds, cloves, and Szechuan peppercorns. Avoid packets of prepared combination seasonings, as well as condiments such as hoisin sauce, mango chutney, and fish sauce. They are usually extremely high in sodium and sometimes high in sugar.

- Add cinnamon to your diet. Recent studies show that cinnamon stimulates circulation and boosts the ability of insulin to metabolize glucose and carry it into cells for energy production.

- Drink water! Drink water! Drink water! I can't stress this enough. Eight to ten 8-ounce glasses a day. You've heard it before. But do it. Water flushes toxins through the kidneys, keeps your body hydrated, and contributes to weight control in several ways: (1) It swells fiber in your stomach. That makes you feel fuller. (2) It reduces fat stores in the body. (3) It cleanses your organs of excess sodium hidden in so many processed foods.

Chapter 10

Exercise

The Secret for People
Who Can't or Won't

Typical scene in a cardiologist's office:

The wife comes in with her husband, the patient.
    She says: "Doctor, can you please make him exercise? I tell
him, but he won't listen. He just won't do it."
    He says: "That's right. I just don't like to exercise."

Cardiologists have long promoted regular exercise to patients because of
the multitude of benefits. Exercise generates energy, burns calories, creates muscle tone, lowers blood pressure, alleviates depression, and lessens
constipation.

    A sedentary lifestyle increases a host of risk factors, which in turn trig-
ger major diseases including CVD. Research shows that just a minimum
amount of some form of activity—a mere thirty minutes a day—yields
major protection, even if you are obese.

    Most of our patients know that. Nevertheless, getting many of
them from point A (knowing it) to point B (doing it) is often very
frustrating.

    If you exercise routinely, you can probably skip this chapter. But if you
are among the 75 percent of adults who fail to get adequate physical

activity and put themselves at increased risk for problems, then stick around. We've got a secret that may get you moving.

Some people function like Popeye after a hit of spinach. They have power, speed, and endurance. Others function more like Popeye before spinach. People definitely demonstrate wide variations in their energy levels and tolerance for exercise.

Recently, researchers from Norway, in conjunction with scientists at the University of Michigan Medical School, turned up some fascinating data that may help explain this basic difference. The investigators found a way to actually breed rats with reduced capacity for aerobic exercise—a kind of "survival of the unfittest" experiment. They essentially bred the weakest rats in each of eleven generations to one another and did the same with the more robust rodents. In all, more than twenty-nine hundred rats were involved.

After eleven generations, the misfit rats, compared to the fitter rats, were found to have a poor concentration of the key mitochondrial proteins needed for energy production and they had high cardiovascular risk factors. By comparison, the rats bred for exercise had healthier mitochondria and sleeker, firmer bodies.

The researchers postulated that impaired function of mitochondria was the underlying metabolic problem in the weaker rats with low aerobic activity levels. The mitochondria, as we have discussed, are the tiny structures within cells that produce ATP to fuel cellular activity. The more impaired the mitochondria, the poorer the inherent skill for and tolerance of physical exercise, and the more probable the animal would have insulin resistance, diabetes, and future cardiovascular disease.

Recent research in humans has also associated poor mitochondrial function with metabolic syndrome, the cluster of risk factors that lead to many health problems, including insulin resistance and type 2 diabetes, high blood pressure, and CVD. The research suggests that if you happen to be genetically endowed with lesser mitochondria, you might be more likely to have a low tolerance for exercise and more prone to develop abdominal fat, diabetes, and cardiovascular problems.

If you don't feel like exercising because it's always been too hard for you, or if you just can't exercise very long before your muscles weaken and you quickly run out of breath, then it could be that you lack some mitochondrial firepower. So stop beating yourself up for being a couch potato. We've got a way to help boost your mitochondria—some magic pills, in fact. Everybody is always looking for those.

Your mitochondria can indeed be fed, fertilized, and fortified.

Although the researchers of the rat study didn't mention it, we can share a big secret based on our years of clinical experience dealing with patients who have profound cardiovascular disease.

The Big Secret: CoQ10, Magnesium, D-ribose, and L-carnitine

We call CoQ10, magnesium, D-ribose, and L-carnitine our awesome foursome because of the way they energize heart muscle cells and the rest of you. We have seen these supplements work like a rocket booster for low-energy patients who never felt like exercising. Research shows, for instance, that D-ribose improves chronic fatigue syndrome because the condition is based on faulty ATP metabolism. CoQ10, L-carnitine, and magnesium also reduce chronic fatigue because they support ATP production. Mice fed CoQ10 practically become mice that roar—more physically active and reproductively potent.

We routinely recommend these mitochondria-nourishing nutrients to generate the energy necessary to physically jumpstart people into exercise. They can transform your mitochondria into the powerhouses they were meant to be.

Previously sedentary patients who start some kind of an activity program, even minimal, consistently tell us they feel better. Exercise and health improvement go hand in hand.

Desire Plus Supplements and He's Back on the Golf Course

Six years ago, Dr. Sinatra met with seventy-eight-year-old Stan and his son. The elderly man was not feeling well. He was taking multiple cardiovascular medications, yet had a poor quality of life. A cardiovascular surgeon had just told Stan's son that Stan's heart was too disabled for a bypass.

Although discouraged, Stan had a powerful desire to get well. Dr. Sinatra recommended that Stan discontinue eight of his twelve drugs and placed him on generous doses of CoQ10, L-carnitine, and magnesium. Stan's health made a complete turnabout. His energy returned. His angina vanished. He participated vigorously in ballroom dancing and in time was playing eighteen holes of golf two to three times a week.

Stan has not taken any nitroglycerin since he started the supplement program six years ago.

In 2005, Stan consulted with another cardiologist, who placed him on Coumadin for atrial fibrillation. However, a subsequent evaluation showed his heart was functioning in regular rhythm.

Since he had no fibrillation, Stan's son, who is a chiropractor, suggested high-dose vitamin E in combination with fish oils to serve as alternative anticoagulants. Dr. Sinatra suggested he also add D-ribose to his supplement program as an additional energy booster.

Stan is a perfect example of a patient who fervently wants to be well, and when the intention of the patient matches the intention of the healer, magnificent things occur. Although Stan was not an exercise shirker, the supplements gave his energy level such a boost that he was able to become happily active again. It never ceases to amaze us how just a few simple supplements can make such a difference in the zest and quality of life of sick patients.

The Bottom Line

If you've been unsuccessful in all your previous attempts at sustained exercise, CoQ10, magnesium, L-carnitine, and D-ribose may be the trick that works for you. The combination doesn't get all our patients into activity, but it works for a lot of them—and they all feel better.

For our dosage suggestions, refer to chapter 12. If you have cardiovascular disease, use the therapeutic dosage recommendations.

Be sure to consult with your physician if you haven't exercised for a long time. Start slowly and build up gradually.

When patients ask us what kind of exercise to do, our answer is always the same: the kind you'll keep doing year after year. Think of something that you enjoy. If you don't like the treadmill but you love to jump rope, then start by jumping rope one minute a day. There are so many things to do; just get yourself up and find something that appeals to you. You don't have to jog a mile a day; just walk your dog around the block. Any activity is better than none, and you may gradually build up your exercise tolerance.

Maybe you can take the stairs instead of the elevator, or park your car a little farther away from your destination. Try to find a way of introducing exercise into your daily activities. You'll be surprised how you can start logging activity minutes just by avoiding some of the common conveniences of modern living.

Join a gym. Join your local hiking club and start taking beginner-level hikes. Try yoga or tai chi. Take morning or evening walks.

There are plenty of books and videos on exercise to guide you. Personal trainers can help you set up an individualized program.

Just start doing something.

Chapter 11

Defusing Stress

*Every stress leaves an indelible scar, and the organism pays for its survival
after a stressful situation by becoming a little older.*
—Hans Selye, M.D.

How Emotion Kills: Dr. Sinatra's Personal Story

When I was thirteen, my paternal grandmother died. She had a massive
stroke and passed away the following day. I felt so sad, and I remember
asking my father what had caused her stroke. He explained that the oil
burner in my grandmother's house had started smoking and she became
emotionally upset about it. Within a few minutes, she became confused.
Then she collapsed to the floor.

I recalled the incident later when I studied the psychological connection to physical disease. I realized that the intense arousal caused by the
smoking oil burner had set the stage for my grandmother to die of an
acute stroke.

While standing at a hospital podium in the mid-1970s and delivering a
lecture on how to prevent heart attacks, the cardiologist Robert S. Eliot
suffered a heart attack. He was forty-four years old.

Eliot survived the event and made a full recovery, during which time he recognized that stress had brought him down. He realized he had to make dramatic lifestyle changes. He was his own first stress patient, as he put it.

With a new lease on life, he went on to establish the Department of Preventive and Stress Medicine at the University of Nebraska Medical Center and to become an outspoken advocate for productivity without self-destruction. In his popular book *Is It Worth Dying For?* Eliot coined the term "FUD factor"—for fear, uncertainty, and doubt. He advised that the best way to handle FUD and stress—particularly intense situations of hostility, anger, and explosive rage—was to be aware that these emotions carry a heavy price, including the potential for sudden death. His mantra was: "Don't sweat the small stuff . . . it's all small stuff, anyway." He was also known for glib phrases such as: "People who smoke together, croak together." We highly recommend his book as a humorous read about a serious subject.

Eliot's title is well taken. Is any emotional event worth dying for? Obviously, no. A short fuse doesn't make for a long life. And if you have high blood pressure to boot, it's important to recognize your vulnerability and explore ways to cope.

For your arteries, stress is like an arsonist with matches in one hand and a gasoline can in the other. You must disarm this perpetrator before he hurts you.

The first thing to realize is that stress is *not what happens to you*—those outside forces are the stressors—but rather *how you react to what happens*. The amount of stress you feel is based on your perception of an event, a person, or a place far more than on the impetus of stress itself. So, when you feel stress, you perceive a threat to your physical or mental well-being that you may or may not be able to respond to adequately.

There is plenty of evidence showing that whenever you address psychological imbalances, such as distressing emotions, anger, and depression, the chances of survival after a cardiovascular event are improved and the risk for having a second event or other health problems is lessened. And, we should add, this obviously applies to prevention as well. People who recognize their emotional issues and find ways to deal with them become less prone to angina, irregular heartbeat, heart attack, stroke, and high blood pressure.

If you have a history of CVD and a nearby hospital or medical center offers a cardiovascular rehabilitation program, it behooves you to join in and use it to work on your risk factors. Some rehab programs deal with only diet and exercise, but the most effective ones include mind/body interventions as well, ranging from yoga and meditation to group support and psychotherapy.

If your hospital program doesn't include a psychosocial component and if your individual needs require it, we advise you to consult a social worker, a psychotherapist, or a counselor who can help you work on your stress and emotional issues. You have many options.

Laugh More

Children laugh an average of 400 times a day. Adults only 15. Somewhere on the way to adulthood, we lose the ability to laugh 385 times a day. This lost ability translates into degrees of reduced physiological function that medical science is now beginning to recognize and quantify, even down to the level of hormones, neurotransmitters, and neuropeptides.

Among the leaders in laughter research is Lee Berk, of Loma Linda University in California. In one study, Berk divided in half a group of cardiac patients who had suffered a heart attack. Both groups received conventional rehabilitation care, but the members in one group also watched a humorous video or sitcom of their choice on a daily basis.

After a year, the data showed that the comedy watchers had significantly lower stress hormone levels and blood pressure readings. They needed fewer medications. They registered healthier electrocardiograph readings. The most profound finding was that among this group there were only two new heart attacks compared to ten in the control group.

At the American College of Cardiology conference in 2005, researchers from the University of Maryland reported that laughter actually makes blood vessels work more efficiently. "Fifteen minutes of laughter on a daily basis is probably good for the vascular system," said the cardiologist Michael Miller.

Miller and his colleagues showed two movies—violent scenes from the 1998 movie *Saving Private Ryan* and the 1996 comedy *King Pin*—to twenty healthy volunteers and then tested the function of their blood vessels. The researchers looked specifically at the endothelium and found that blood flow was reduced in fourteen of the twenty volunteers after viewing stressful clips. But blood flowed more freely in nineteen of the twenty when they laughed at funny movie segments. Average blood flow increased 22 percent during laughter and decreased 35 percent during mental stress.

"The endothelium is the first line in the development of atherosclerosis, so, given the results of our study, it is conceivable that laughing may be important to maintain a healthy endothelium and reduce the risk of cardiovascular disease," Miller said.

In a second study presented at the forum, Wei Jiang, of Duke University, reported on the other side of the emotional coin: depression. The researchers followed 1,005 heart failure patients and also tested them for depression. The ones with mild depression had a 44 percent greater risk of dying, according to the study.

"Approximately half of all patients with heart failure die within five years of diagnosis, and we believe that our study appears to identify a group of these patients who are at a higher risk for dying," Jiang said. It was not clear why, but patients with depression tend to exercise less, smoke more, eat poorly, and not take medications properly.

The obvious lesson here: find something that makes you laugh—a lot.

Give and Receive Affection

Do you feel loved? Are you happily married? These factors make a difference in your cardiovascular health.

Research shows that marital status is a prime factor in the recovery and longevity of men following a heart attack. Those who fare the best and live longer tend to feel that their wives love them, while those with poorer survival records tend to feel unloved.

The marital effect on men has been known for quite a while, but only recently did a group of researchers at San Diego State University find strong evidence that it's the same for women. In a fascinating study published in 2003, the investigators assessed carotid and coronary artery health, along with cardiovascular risk factors, in 393 women. These assessments, including ultrasound and electron beam tomography, were made at the beginning of the study and then eleven to fourteen years later. Women in satisfying marriages had the least atherosclerosis and also tended to show less rapid progression of carotid disease compared to individuals in low-satisfying marriages. Women without partners had intermediate levels of artery degeneration. The researchers concluded that a high-quality marriage may protect against cardiovascular disease for women.

In a study of 165 patients undergoing angiograms at the Yale University School of Medicine, individuals who felt loved and supported had less coronary artery disease.

Obviously, affection serves the heart well. And not just in humans, as was realized from an Ohio State cholesterol study conducted with rabbits in the 1970s. Several groups of animals were fed extremely high-cholesterol diets, and, with the exception of one group, all developed artery-clogging heart disease. The animals that deviated from the norm had 60 percent fewer symptoms. The puzzled researchers could not account for this result until they discovered by chance that the student in charge of feeding this particular group of rabbits enjoyed cuddling and fondling each animal before feeding it. The isolation itself was atherogenic, while the caring and cuddling was protective.

Meditation

Meditation has been around for thousands of years, but it clearly has major therapeutic merit for combating modern stress and contemporary disease such as CVD.

Many forms of meditation exist. You simply need to find one that works for you and do it regularly. Continuity generates maximum benefits for the nervous system usually running at full steam ahead.

The relaxation response, an offshoot of traditional meditation, was developed at Harvard in the 1970s by the cardiologist Herbert Benson as a way to deflate stress-induced high blood pressure. Benson showed he could produce a protective mechanism against stress, something opposite of the fight-or-flight response. To achieve the relaxation response, you repeat a simple, neutral word, such as *one*, for several minutes.

Over the years, Benson noted even more profound physiological changes by incorporating what he terms the *faith factor*. That means repeating a simple prayer or statement reflecting spiritual roots or beliefs. For example, using phrases like *The Lord is my shepherd* or *Hail Mary, full of grace*, or words like *shalom* or *om*. After you choose your phrase, you simply close your eyes and breathe in through your nose. You say your word or phrase silently as you exhale. When stray thoughts come by, gently release them and continue your phrase. Use this technique for ten to fifteen minutes once or twice a day.

Transcendental meditation (TM), a method exported from India's Himalayas by Maharishi Mahesh Yogi in 1957, is the most thoroughly researched form of meditation. To date, more than five hundred studies have been done, including $20 million worth of major ongoing investigations on blood pressure funded by the National Institutes of Health. The studies show that TM lowers high blood pressure as significantly as conventional treatments and medication but without side effects.

Transcendental meditation is a simple and natural mental technique taught worldwide that anyone can learn, but you need a trained instructor to teach you (call 888-532-7686 or visit www.tm.org). It is practiced for twenty minutes twice a day and does not involve any religious belief, philosophy, or change in lifestyle. During TM, the thinking process effortlessly settles down until mental activity of ordinary waking consciousness is "transcended" and a unique state of restful alertness is created. In addition, there is a corresponding settling down of the body's machinery.

Studies indicate that transcending and a resultant deep physiological rest offer a powerful natural antidote to chronic stress and other major risk factors for CVD. The documented benefits include reduced blood pressure, reduced use of tobacco and alcohol, lowering of high cholesterol and lipid oxidation, and decreased psychosocial stress. Recently, researchers found that four months of meditation significantly improved the ability of arterial endothelium to relax and dilate. The changes resulting from these effects include improvement of atherosclerosis, reduction of myocardial ischemia and left ventricular hypertrophy, reduced health insurance claims for CVD, and reduced mortality.

Meditation Plus

Meditation is a cornerstone of the Program for Reversing Heart Disease developed by Dean Ornish, director of the Preventive Medicine Research Institute in Sausalito, California, and a clinical professor of medicine at the University of California, San Francisco. Ornish's program, featured in books and widely publicized in the media, also includes a low-fat vegetarian diet, moderate regular exercise, yoga, smoke cessation, and participation in professionally supervised support group sessions.

"People are able to eliminate the symptoms of coronary heart disease and become functionally normal," said Ornish. "We have proven that intensive lifestyle modification alone can dramatically improve patients with moderate to severe disease without costly operations or a lifetime of cholesterol-lowering drugs."

Originally ridiculed by his conservative peers for what was considered an off-the-wall idea, Ornish followed his convictions and went on to document for the first time that coronary artery disease could be reversed by lifestyle. In his series of studies published in leading medical journals, Ornish compared the results of patients following his program with others receiving usual and customary care. In regard to chest pain, his patients as a group attained reductions of 91 percent in frequency, 42 percent in duration, and 38 percent in severity. Patients in the comparison group experienced symptoms of worsening disease.

Of keen interest to scientists was the actual determination—through sophisticated cardiology imaging techniques—of reversal of blocked arterial tissue among program participants. The exciting proof was first reported in 1990.

The way to picture this is to imagine the narrowest points of blockage in the arteries beginning to open up. Previous studies involving medication showed that blockages could be widened, but to a much smaller degree.

In September 1995, additional evidence was published demonstrating that patients in the program for five years had significantly improved blood flow to the heart muscle. It is well and good to improve the artery, but if you can't improve the flow, it doesn't mean anything. The new findings showed improvement to both. Some 99 percent of Ornish's patients showed improvement against 45 percent in the comparison group receiving standard care.

Unlike other rehabilitative programs, the Ornish method strongly addressed the anxiety, anger, depression, and social isolation associated with heart disease through group sessions and stress management techniques that include meditation, visualization, progressive relaxation, and yoga (stretching) performed for more than an hour a day. For more information on this program, refer to his book, *Dr. Dean Ornish's Program for Reversing Heart Disease*, or go online to www.ornish.com.

Faith

Religious belief, affiliation, and practices are associated with better health, better health outcomes following illness, and longevity. As an example, researchers at Johns Hopkins University partnered with sixteen Baltimore churches to investigate the impact of various nutrition and physical activity strategies on African American women aged forty and over. The big winner, after a year, was the on-site program at churches. Compared to a self-help group that registered little gain, the church-based group made significant inroads in weight loss, blood pressure, and waist girth reduction.

"Urban African American women over forty bear a marked excess risk of obesity and death from heart disease," commented Diane M. Becker, director of the Johns Hopkins Center for Health Promotion. "This study demonstrates that church-based interventions can greatly improve their cardiovascular health."

Magnesium: The Antistress Mineral

We discussed magnesium earlier (chapter 6) and how it relaxes arteries, lowers blood pressure, and promotes cellular energy. We reintroduce this vital mineral again in the context of its totally overlooked importance in counteracting stress.

Stress can kill. But stress, along with magnesium deficiency, is even deadlier. The combination is a serious yet unheralded cause of death and suffering in the United States, concluded Mildred Seelig, an Emory University professor of family and preventive medicine, after decades of research.

According to Seelig, "Magnesium deficiency intensifies adverse reactions to stress that can be not only life-threatening but life-ending. All stress and trauma, whether physical or emotional, causes a loss of the body's stores of magnesium. And if you don't have enough magnesium to begin with, you run the risk of more serious reactions."

The typical magnesium-deficient American diet produces little magnesium for the body to store, so stress may quickly put you into the red.

"In essence, you are creating a second front of stress, and thus you have intensification of stress reactions," Seelig contended. "Without adequate magnesium and the life-supporting activities it contributes to in the body, events can dramatically become life-threatening."

Medically, perhaps the most dramatic evidence of the stress-magnesium connection concerns cardiovascular disease. Magnesium deficiency increases the risk of hypertension, cerebrovascular and coronary artery constriction and occlusion, arrhythmias, and sudden cardiac death.

Attitude

If you have CVD, please check your attitude. We're not joking. Patients have to want to heal. Seneca, the Roman playwright, put it succinctly two thousand years ago when he said, "It is part of the cure to wish to be cured."

Much closer to our time, researchers were amazed to find that CVD patients who took at least 80 percent of their placebo pills during a five-year controlled study on cholesterol reduction had a mortality rate similar to those who took the active medication. In the experiment, some eleven hundred men were randomly divided to take either the placebo or the drug. The subjects didn't know if the pill they took was for real or fake. Among the most zealous compliers in both categories (who we assume believed they were taking something that might make them better), there was a similar 15 percent mortality rate. Among the more lax followers, the rate was 25 percent in those assigned to the medication and 28 percent for placebo takers. It's amazing what attitude can do.

Even with our basic medical education and specialization training, patients teach doctors a great deal. They change and inspire us, especially when we encounter individuals who, by their own personal strength, intuition, and character, are able to endure and thrive despite extreme physical difficulties and the constrictions of "official" medicine.

One such person was Fran, who came to one of us (Dr. Sinatra) in her quest for a "health coach" to assist her with an expanded self-care program. Fran believed that a positive attitude was central to self-healing. She also knew intuitively that she had the ability to help heal her own heart. Unfortunately, her conventional doctors disagreed and discouraged her. There was nothing she could do on her own that would be of any real help, they asserted. They told her to stick to the medication, and if her condition deteriorated, a heart transplant was her only option.

Although frustrated, stressed, despondent, and discouraged, Fran believed that her improvement depended on an integrated approach including vitamin and mineral therapy, some kind of relaxation technique, psychotherapy, energy work, and acupuncture in addition to conventional medicine. She asked for guidance.

Fran wanted to know about targeted natural healing therapies and nutritional supplements as well as positive affirmations and mental imagery. She followed the advice she received, and she got better. She needed less medication and avoided a heart transplant.

Fran's search for physical, emotional, and spiritual support is the best approach to healing. Over many years of medical practice, we have both learned that the most important way to help someone overcome a disease is to help them stimulate and nurture their own inner resources, "the doctor within," as some people refer to it. This often boosts recovery in a powerful way.

Healing is not just taking a "magic" pill. Patients' symptoms may get better, but they won't be healthier. Getting and staying well involves working on the physical, emotional, and spiritual level. That's when "miracles" occur. Self-healing enables the awesome process to unfold. Thorough healing often encompasses both conventional and nonconventional therapies.

We've learned that as resistant as some patients are to improving their lifestyle and health habits, others are equally as resistant not to give in to disease and death sentences. We've worked with countless patients who simply refused to throw in the towel when multiple doctors told them that they had a limited time to live. Instead, they dug in, became actively involved in their recoveries, and got well. It's absolutely amazing what the spirit can overcome! These patients wanted to live. When you have that kind of resolve and willingness to educate yourself and make the necessary changes so that your body can heal, incredible recoveries can and do happen.

The American Heart Association Recommendations

The American Heart Association offers an array of strategies for reducing stress, particularly if you have CVD. They include:

- Talk with family, friends, clergy, or other trusted advisers about your concerns and stresses, and ask for their support.

- Learn to accept things you can't change. You don't have to solve all of life's problems.

- Count to ten before answering or responding when you feel angry.

- Don't use smoking, drinking, overeating, drugs, or caffeine to cope with stress. They make things worse.

- Look for the good in situations instead of the bad.

- Exercise regularly. Do something you enjoy, such as swimming, jogging, golfing, walking a pet, tai chi, or cycling. Check with your doctor to determine what activity level is right for you.

- Be an animal caregiver. Elderly individuals with animal companions make fewer visits to doctors than nonowners and do much better following heart attacks. They have better blood pressure numbers.

- Think ahead about what may upset you and try to avoid it. For example, spend less time with people who bother you. Adjust your schedule to avoid driving in rush-hour traffic.

- Plan productive solutions to problems. For example, talk with your neighbor if the dog next door bothers you. Set clear limits on how much you'll do for family members.

- Learn to say no. Don't promise too much. Give yourself enough time to get things done.

- Join a support group—maybe for people with heart disease, for women, for men, for retired persons, or some other group with which you identify.

And one more thing: practice altruism. The Bible reminds us that it's more blessed to give than to receive. By giving, we don't necessarily mean money but kind deeds that help the lives of others. While they feel the generosity, science indicates that the giver receives the biggest dividend.

Researchers at the University of Michigan found that giving actually promotes longevity. Receiving, by contrast, had no such effect. They reached this conclusion based on a ten-year follow-up of three thousand men. The individuals who did volunteer work just once a week were two and a half times less likely to die during that period than those who did not volunteer. Ninety-five percent of the volunteer group said that helping others on a regular, personal basis gave them a physical sensation or warmth, increased energy, and euphoria—the so-called helper's high.

Helping others helps you. It reduces stress, increases happiness, decreases depression, and improves both mental and physical health. It generates a sense of belonging, of mattering. These positive gains are good for the body, the immune system, cardiovascular health, and a longer life.

Chapter 12

Putting It All Together
The New Cardiology Unclog Program

A 2003 study in the *Journal of Medical Genetics* on seventy-two men who had reached the age of a hundred revealed that they had higher levels of anti-inflammatory substances in the body than men of other age groups. The message: keep your anti-inflammatory defenses strong and you will live a longer life. This chapter will give you the specific New Cardiology guidelines.

Obviously, the best way to start a New Cardiology program is to visit with doctors like us for a personalized program. If you are interested, you'll find a list of integrative cardiologists in appendix A.

If that's not a practical option, read on and follow the general game plan that we have developed. It is based on treating thousands of patients. The program has four major elements—the four pillars of healing. Adopt them in a way that's comfortable for you if you have had a stroke, heart

---

If You Have CVD

If you have symptoms such as chest pain, shortness of breath, or difficulty walking, see your doctor immediately. Our suggestions may be helpful, but it is more vital that you obtain immediate medical attention. Your life may depend on it.

---

attack, bypass surgery, stent procedures, angioplasty, or suffer with heart failure. *But be sure to consult with your doctor before trying any of our recommendations.*

The Four Pillars of Healing

PILLAR 1

- An anti-inflammatory diet.
- Good weight management. A trimmer body is better for a compromised heart. A healthy diet and carefully paced exercise can help you reach a *healthy* weight.
- Don't ignore your oral hygiene. Bacteria from periodontal disease can stir up the flames of arterial disease. Later in the chapter, we'll make some simple but effective recommendations.

PILLAR 2

- Targeted nutritional supplements (see our guidelines in this chapter on how to create your individual program).
- Medication therapy, as required and individualized for the patient.

PILLAR 3

- Exercise. For individuals with angina, heart failure, and peripheral artery disease, be sure to get out and walk. But listen to your body. Stop if you develop shortness of breath, chest pain, or cramping of the legs. Symptomatic patients need to scale down their exercise. Your physician may wish to carry out a treadmill exam to give you an exercise prescription. We strongly advise any patient undergoing bypass surgery or who has had a heart attack to join a supervised cardiac rehabilitation program to learn how to identify bodily sensations when exercising. We believe that a major purpose of cardiac rehab is to get you in touch with your body. Call your local hospital for information on such programs.

PILLAR 4

- Mind/body techniques. People with cardiovascular disease sometimes develop mood disorders. Following an event or surgery, depression may occur for six months to a year, or what we call postpump syndrome associated with confusion and mental impairment.

If you or someone in your family recognizes a change in mood or mental function, be sure to seek out specialized care. Consult with your doctor. Support groups can be very helpful for these situations.

Be keenly aware of the danger of anger and stress (see chapter 11) that can trigger major cardiovascular events. If you have a temper problem, you may need to work with a coach or a specific guided program.

Does the Integrative Approach Really Work?

You bet it does. As clinicians seeking the very best outcome for our patients, we are not in the position to do formal research in which you put one group of patients on one program and compare them to another group that takes a placebo pill or does something different. We simply couldn't deny some of our patients the recommendations that we know to be effective. So if you are wondering whether our program and specifically the supplements we suggest have been researched collectively, the answer is no. However, the individual supplements have vast scientific support. We base our strategies on all of those many individual studies and our own clinical experience in putting all the elements together.

One example of how well such comprehensive approaches work was demonstrated at the Alfred Hospital and Baker Heart Research Institute in Melbourne, Australia. The cardiologist Franklin Rosenfeldt and his colleagues wanted to monitor a combined supplement/physical exercise/mental stress–reduction program on patients with aging hearts who have a lesser ability to withstand and recover from different kinds of stress. Their supplement program featured CoQ10, alpha-lipoic acid, magnesium, and omega-3 fatty acids. The combined therapy, they found, effectively sped recovery time.

In another experiment, Rosenfeldt's group started sixteen heart patients on a similar program about a month before cardiac surgery. Six weeks after surgery, they found the patients experienced significant improvements in medical tests and quality of life compared to other patients receiving conventional care. The Australian researchers concluded that a program of "combined metabolic, physical, and mental preparation before cardiac surgery is safe, feasible, and may improve quality of life, lower systolic blood pressure, reduce levels of oxidative stress, and thus has the potential to enhance postoperative recovery."

Among our patients, we consistently see significant recoveries and improvement. Here are two examples.

Doug

Literally at death's door, sixty-three-year-old Doug had severe coronary artery disease. He refused bypass surgery because he is a self-employed shopowner and couldn't afford to be out of commission during the two-month recovery period. As a veteran, the bypass would have been free for him.

Doug experienced a minor heart attack in 2001. Two arteries were stented. Chest pains recurred the next summer. His cardiologist performed an angiogram. The test showed 60 percent narrowing in the left main coronary artery, thus compromising blood flow to two-thirds of the heart muscle. Two other arteries contained significant narrowings and a third had closed.

Any cardiologist would recommend bypass for a patient in this serious shape. Doug refused and came to Dr. Roberts instead.

He complained of chest pain at rest, even with medication. He was already on a statin to lower cholesterol. He was tested for New Cardiology risk factors and had them aplenty: elevated fibrinogen, homocysteine, an off-the-chart Lp(a) of 93, lead and mercury, insulin resistance, and low free testosterone.

Doug still refused bypass. He was then started on a supplement program, including CoQ10, L-carnitine, antioxidants and minerals, nanobacteria therapy, and heavy metal detoxification. Later on, L-arginine and pellet testosterone therapy were added.

Doug's symptoms disappeared. His HDL went up and LDL went down.

Less than a year later, he was able to walk nine minutes on the tread-mill. It took him five minutes before he started to develop chest pain. Without informing Dr. Roberts, Doug stopped all his anti-anginal drugs. He didn't miss them.

The next winter Doug vacationed in St. Augustine, Florida. While there, he climbed to the top of the landmark lighthouse. A companion tired and had to stop halfway up.

Doug's stress study was repeated in early 2005, three and a half years into his treatment program. He walked for ten minutes. Chest pain didn't occur until six minutes. This represents a phenomenal improvement in functional capacity and a good outlook for Doug. We view treadmill time as a big decision maker. If you can walk for ten minutes, you are not likely to die. If you have to stop at two minutes, you have a big functional problem. Pretreatment, Doug experienced pain at rest!

An operation was called for in Doug's case, but he wouldn't go for it. So he got the alternative side of New Cardiology alone. It worked, and he's feeling great.

James

James, seventy-one, was taking CoQ10 and other antioxidants but was not showing expected progress. He had a totally blocked right coronary artery, along with some nonsevere blockage in the other coronary arteries. The heart muscle was being fed in part by natural collateral bypasses. He was having pain at rest.

Dr. Sinatra added L-arginine. Two weeks later, James's pain went away. We didn't have to change his anatomy by opening up a blocked artery. In his case, it was sufficient just to change the physiology of his blood flow with a common and inexpensive amino acid supplement you can buy at the health food store. It dilated his arteries and improved blood flow so that his heart got more oxygen and nutrients.

James exercises now and can perform many more activities than he could do before. Conventional medicine might have called for a single-vessel bypass. Here he got an added supplement—just what his body needed.

Sometimes you can give a patient two or three elements in the program and nothing seems to happen. Then you can add one more and like magic that seems to carry the patient into a new healing dimension.

Putting Together a Therapeutic Supplement Program

In chapters 6 and 7, we reviewed many nutritional supplements that can make a big difference in the life of a CVD patient. Those supplements counteract inflammation and stabilize plaque . . . and in some cases even reverse plaque. We have listed them here. Check back to those earlier chapters for our detailed recommendations and to be sure that the supplement and dosage are appropriate for you.

Admittedly, this is a long list. However, CVD is no lightweight disease. And if it is well advanced, you need all the supplement firepower you can muster to overcome it.

Supplement	Your Daily Dosage	Comments
Multivitamin/mineral with antioxidants	Follow label instructions.	The most effective multiformulas require that you take several or more capsules/tablets daily.
Fish oil	2–4 g	Be sure the product you take is pharmaceutical grade—that is, free of contaminants. The label will tell you.
Magnesium	400–800 mg	
CoQ10	100–300 mg or more	See chapter 7 for dosage and form specifics.
L-carnitine	1–3 g	Take half the recommended dosage if you have a stable heart—that is, no heart failure.
D-ribose	10–15 g	Take half the recommended dosage if you don't have heart failure or angina.
L-arginine	6–8 g	
DetoxMaxPlus: phosphatidylcholine (essential phospholipids) with EDTA	1 oz twice a week	Available through doctors only. See chapters 6 and 8.
Nattokinase and lumbrokinase	Nattokinase: 4,000 units a day. For strokes, 6,000 units. Lumbrokinase: Two 20 mg capsules thirty minutes before meals, three times daily for four weeks. Then one capsule three times daily.	You can omit these supplements if you do not have toxic blood, indicated by elevated homocysteine, fibrinogen, and Lp(a), which put you at higher risk for clotting.
Vitamin C	At least 1,000 mg	

Supplement	Your Daily Dosage	Comments
B-complex vitamins		Usually a multi contains enough of the B-complex factors. You may need to take extra folic acid, vitamin B-6, and vitamin B-12 if you have elevated homocysteine. Take extra niacin if you have low HDL.
Vitamin E	200 IU	A multi usually has vitamin E in it, but we recommend you take a full-spectrum vitamin E supplement containing mixed tocopherols, preferably with tocotrienols.
Garlic	1,000 mg	We recommend high-allicin forms.
Vitamin K-2	150 mcg	Available in early 2007 in health food stores and online at www.drsinatra.com.

Optional
  L-lysine
  L-proline
	
	2,000 mg twice daily
	1,000 mg twice daily
		For individuals with high Lp(a), rapid disease progress and blockages, and repeated cardiovascular events. Lp(a) does not come down in blood tests, but patients improve dramatically.

How to Take Supplements

Start your supplement program slowly. Begin with one supplement and slowly add in the others. Depending on what you take, you could phase in your program along these lines:

Phase 1: a multivitamin supplement (containing antioxidants), vitamin C, and fish oil

Phase 2: CoQ10, L-carnitine, D-ribose, magnesium, and vitamin K-2

Phase 3: L-arginine, garlic, and, if indicated, the detox supplement

Take your multivitamin/antioxidants and fish oil with meals. The antioxidants blunt the rise in CRP and clotting factors that otherwise accompany sugar and fat intake.

Amino acids (such as L-carnitine and L-arginine) and clot digesters (such as nattokinase and lumbrokinase) work better if taken between meals or at least thirty minutes before eating.

In the big picture, timing is not so critical. It is more important for you to take what you need and stay with the program. If you stop the supplements, you lose the benefits. If you have a hectic schedule, take the supplements whenever you can. Find the schedule that works for you.

If you happen to develop a reaction to a particular supplement, change the time of day you take it or take it with a meal. If you know the problem is with a specific supplement, you may want to change brands.

How Can You Tell If the Program Is Working?

Obviously, objective medical tests, such as ejection fraction and treadmills, can document progress. But you'll know simply from your own experience. The program is working for you if

- You need to take less nitroglycerin or even none at all

What Our Patients Tell Us

Patients on the New Cardiology program enthusiastically tell us they feel better and are more satisfied with the quality of their lives. They show more interest in others. One patient said that after having the black cloud removed from over his head, he was participating more in his family life. He bought his wife flowers. He got more involved in his son's school activities.

The most important thing is how you feel. If the treadmill time doesn't improve but your quality of life improves and you have less pain, we are gratified as doctors. When patients start joking, we know they are mending.

- Your previous chest pain decreases or even disappears
- Your breathing improves and you have less shortness of breath
- You can perform daily activities with less discomfort or impairment
- You have more energy
- You sleep better
- Your relationships are better
- You feel more joy and gratitude at having a second chance at life

How Much Will All This Cost?

Fair question. We get it all the time from our patients.

We have recommended supplements for many years—five decades between us—and are very sensitive to the issue of cost. Unfortunately, some supplements are expensive, and collectively you could be looking at up to several hundred dollars a month.

Moreover, don't look to your insurance company to help you. Because of the distorted nature of our medical system, insurance will pay tens of thousands of dollars for hospital procedures to patch you up but won't pay a few hundred dollars for supplements to keep you *out* of the hospital. If you can figure the logic in that, please let us know.

Our program emphasizes personal responsibility. Your health is priceless, but to raise your health from poor to good, you have to pay a price both in effort and money. By not changing your lifestyle, you are pretty much stuck. The medical system may fix you up when you get into trouble, but you're the one who has to do the work to stay out of subsequent trouble. Don't count on the system to make you healthier.

We see copayments for prescriptions rising and even insurance plans not covering a lot of medications. We are concerned that as health care resources become increasingly strained with the aging of baby boomers, patients may not be able to get a fully covered bypass in fifteen years, maybe not in five years. You can't rely on Medicare to take care of you. You have to spend some personal resources now to avoid spending huge dollars in the future. If you were to take five or so drugs, you might spend $250 a month, anyway. Not only do you bear the cost but also the potential of side effects. Why not spend some money now to get healthier—and you may not have to deal with serious crises in the future.

We've treated many patients who thought they were going to be taken care of by their insurance companies and weren't. So you need to do all you can to become healthier and not get sick. This program can help you do that. It's like a retirement plan for your health.

Sometimes new patients come in toting shopping bags full of supplement bottles. They will ask which ones they need. Not infrequently, they are spending $400 to $600 a month on supplements and not getting the desired results.

For us it's a matter of getting the most for your money. Our supplement program isn't cheap, but it's effective. And not infrequently, our recommendations cost less money than what a new patient is already spending. We figure the costs as follows:

Supplement	Approximate Cost per Month
Multivitamins/minerals, including B vitamins and antioxidants	$25
Niacin (vitamin B-3)	$15
Fish oil	$20
Magnesium	$15
CoQ10	$40
L-carnitine	$25
D-ribose	$40
L-arginine	$15 in bulk
Nattokinase	$25
Vitamin C	$10
Vitamin E	$15 (if separate from a multivitamin)
Vitamin K-2	$20
Total	$265
Optional:	
Essential phospholipids with EDTA	$200 per month for the first year; $50 per month for the second year and beyond
Bioidentical testosterone	$10–80, depending on form
L-lysine	$20
L-proline	$10

Is There a Bare-Bones Supplement Program?

Some of our Medicare patients simply don't have the resources for a full supplement program. They ask if we have a minimum effective program. If you have CVD and can't afford the entire program, at least take the following:

Supplement	Approximate Cost per Month
Multivitamins/minerals with B vitamins and antioxidants	$25
Fish oil	$20
Magnesium	$15
CoQ10	$25–$40
Vitamin C	$10
Total	$95–$110

Too Far Gone?

Some individuals with advanced atherosclerosis have plaque buildup considered too far gone for standard medicine. In New Cardiology, we try to stabilize blockages and improve blood flow to the heart with innovative approaches. One is EECP—enhanced external counterpulsation—which restores the flow of oxygenated blood in patients with recurrent or inoperable coronary disease. EECP works by placing large blood pressure cufflike devices around the legs and lower half of a patient's body. The cuffs inflate and deflate in rhythm with the heartbeat to push blood from the lower extremities back to the heart, improving flow to the coronary arteries and encouraging the formation of collateral vessels. Think of collateral vessels as natural bypasses. EECP doesn't remove plaque, but it improves blood flow to the oxygen-starved heart. This outpatient, negligible risk therapy is covered by Medicare and most insurers. There are more than a thousand medical clinics using this technology. Dr. Roberts has treated more than eight hundred patients with EECP during the past eight years. For more information on this method, visit his Web site at www.heartfixer.com.

For patients even too far gone for EECP, Dr. Roberts and a group of colleagues are researching the use of magnetic molecular energizer (MME) therapy. In MME, a powerful static magnetic field is applied to the heart. The rate of electron spin around the nucleus of atoms increases, speeding up all useful biochemical reactions in the heart, including ATP energy production and utilization. Stem cells within the heart are stimulated to proliferate and differentiate into replacement cells. Multiple improvements result: better blood flow, healthier blood vessels, the ability of the heart to pump and relax, increased ejection fraction (which sometimes even normalizes), returned function in areas previously scarred by heart attack, and reduced angina and shortness of breath. This exciting technique also benefits disease states involving other internal organs, such as improving functional status in children with cerebral palsy and adults with spinal cord injury. For more on MME and where it is available, visit the Web site www.amri-ohio.com.

Abnormal Test Results

In chapter 4, we listed our healthy zone values for CVD-related blood tests. If any of your results are out of the healthy zone, we offer the following suggestions for specific supplements and lifestyle remedies.

Some of the New Cardiology remedies are covered by insurance and others are not. Some may require a prescription. If you are under medical supervision, please check with your physician before following any of these suggestions. Unless otherwise noted, dosages are daily recommendations.

What You Can Do to Normalize Abnormal Scores

Blood Component	Your Level	Healthy Zone	Interventions That Work for Us
CoQ10	_____	1.0–1.8 µg/ml	Hydrosoluble CoQ10, 30–60 mg. Therapeutic dosages are higher. See the footnote for targeted blood levels when illness is present.
CRP	_____	<0.8 mg/L	Statin drugs. Exercise. Low-dose aspirin. Fish oil, 2 g. Antioxidants. Nattokinase, 2,000 units. Hydrosoluble CoQ10, 30–60 mg.

Blood Component	Your Level	Healthy Zone	Interventions That Work for Us
Ferritin (iron)	_____	Women <80 µg/L	If more than 100 µg/L, donate blood one to three
	_____	Men <90 µg/L	times a year. Do not take more than 500 mg of vitamin C per day until your ferritin level has decreased. If your level is more than 400, ask your doctor to check you for genetic hemochromatosis.
Fibrinogen	_____	180–350 mg/dl	Fish oil, 1–2 g. Garlic or bromelain, 500–1,000 mg. Drink ginger and/or green tea. Lumbrokinase or nattokinase.
Homocysteine	_____	<9 µmol/L	Folic acid, 800 mcg. Vitamin B-6, 40 mg. Vitamin B-12, 200 mcg. Trimethylglycine, 1,000 mg. For individuals with genetic defects in folic acid metabolism, use Metafolin, a patented and highly absorbable form of folic acid (see supplement section in appendix A). Eat more beets and broccoli.
Lp(a)	_____	<30 mg/dl	Niacin, 250–500 mg three to four times daily (may cause flushing). Vitamin C, 500–1,000 mg or more. Fish oil, 1–2 g. Avoid foods with trans-fatty acids. Women: Consider natural estrogen. Men: Avoid soy, and consider testosterone. Bioidentical estrogen and testosterone lower Lp(a).

Blood Component	Your Level	Healthy Zone	Interventions That Work for Us
Total cholesterol	_____	125–200 mg/dl	Reduce weight. Exercise. Increase fiber in diet. Eat soy products, oats, and oatmeal. Chromium, 200 mcg. Hydro-soluble CoQ10, 90–120 mg. Tocotrienol (a form of vitamin E), 50–100 mg. Garlic, 400–800 mg. Plant sterols (phytosterols), 500–1,500 mg. Probiotics (healthy bacteria supplement). Red yeast rice extract, 1,200 mg twice daily. Flax, 2 tbsp crushed flaxseed a day in a healthy shake with 8 oz. soy milk or sprinkled on cereal or salad as a source of fiber. Promotes bowel movements that carry cholesterol out of the body.
HDL	_____ _____	Women 40–120 mg/dl Men 35–70 mg/dl	Assess for insulin resistance if low. Reduce weight. Exercise. Eat fewer high-glycemic carbohydrates. Niacin, 500–1,000 mg. L-carnitine, 500–1,000 mg.
LDL	_____	70–130 mg/dl	See Total cholesterol. LDL greater than 130 in presence of documented coronary artery disease indicates that statin therapy needed.
Oxidized LDL	_____	0–650 units	Elevated oxidized LDL, along with high fibrinogen and CRP, indicates the presence of an advanced inflammatory process. If this is the case, initiate interventions to reduce inflammation. We recommend statin therapy with fish oil, 2 g, and a program of

Blood Component	Your Level	Healthy Zone	Interventions That Work for Us
Oxidized LDL (cont'd)			antioxidants. Exercise and stress management are essential. Follow up with your physician to assess progress.
Triglycerides	_____	50–180 ml/dl	Weight reduction. Exercise. Restrict carbohydrates. Fish oil, 2–3 g. L-carnitine, 1–2 g. Reduce alcohol intake.
AA/EPA ratio	_____	1.5–3	A score greater than 3 indicates the presence of inflammation. The higher the number, the more inflammation. If your omega-6 to omega-3 fatty acid ratio is too high, as reflected by the levels of arachidonic (AA) and eicosapentaenoic (EPA) fatty acids, there's not enough anti-inflammatory EPA in the body to neutralize the proinflammatory AA. We see very unhealthy scores, sometimes as high as 20. Follow the diet suggestions in chapter 9. Also, take 2–3 g of fish oil daily to help neutralize inflammation. In some cases, more may be needed.

Tests for Insulin Resistance

| Fasting blood sugar | _____ | <100 mg/dl | Weight loss. Exercise. Restrict carbohydrates, especially sugary high-glycemic carbs (see appendix B). Use lower-glycemic carbohydrates, such as broccoli, chickpeas, and lentils, to lower insulin levels. |

Blood Component	Your Level	Healthy Zone	Interventions That Work for Us
Fasting blood sugar (cont'd)			Specific supplements: alpha-lipoic acid, 100–300 mg; hydrosoluble CoQ10, 60–90 mg; cinnamon, 1,000 mg; gymnema leaf extract, 200–400 mg; magnesium, 400–800 mg; chromium pico-linate, 100–200 mcg.
Fasting insulin	_____	<17 µg/L	See Fasting blood sugar.
Hemoglobin A1C	_____	<6% of total HGB	See Fasting blood sugar. If weight reduction, exercise, and supplements do not improve percentage, consider pharmaceutical therapy. Ask your physician about Met-formin, a glucose-lowering medication.

Aim to reach or improve these CoQ10 blood levels when the following medical conditions are present:

2.0–2.5 µg/ml	High blood pressure, mitral valve prolapse (MVP), arrhythmia, diabetes, or periodontal disease
2.5–3.5 µg /ml	Mild to moderate heart failure, chronic fatigue syndrome, or angina
>3.5 µg /ml	Severe heart failure

Heart Attack Prevention

People usually consult with a cardiologist when their primary physician refers them following an event, if they have symptoms, or if a test indicates a cardiovascular problem. Many times, a cardiologist has first contact with a patient in a hospital emergency room or an intensive care unit.

Increasingly, we see patients interested in prevention, but still relatively few by comparison to the number of patients who see us with a problem. We hope this trend grows. We feel that with today's sophisticated diagnostics we can effectively predict problems before they arise and recommend simple interventions—as easy as taking a few supplements a day—to deter and head off arterial inflammation. And because we view inflammation as a marker of premature aging, preventive screening for cardiovascular status can double as a test for accelerated aging in general.

When we are out lecturing, many people ask us what kind of testing we recommend so that they can then ask their own physicians. Please refer to chapter 4 for those details.

We constantly drill into the heads of our patients the importance of taking responsibility for their own health. That's what prevention is all about: what *you* do to make yourself healthier. We can prescribe pills, supplements, and sophisticated tests, dole out advice, and send you to surgery if you need it, but what you do 24/7 makes the biggest difference.

After treating thousands of patients with the gravest of conditions, we can tell you unequivocally that prevention is a whole lot easier on you (and us) than treatment. The research suggests that many of us already have plaque formation brewing by the time we hit adulthood. That's why we believe it makes good sense to adopt a prevention attitude as early as possible. Financial planners tell you to start investing for your retirement early. Obviously, retirement based on financial security is wonderful. But if you don't have the good health to go along with it, you are not going to enjoy the fruits of your labor. If you want a retirement with good health, you need to start working early on your health, just as you do on your finances. Don't wait until you get sick.

Prevention is not complicated. Our four pillars of healing that we laid out earlier in this chapter are important. As far as supplements are concerned, you don't need as many as someone with CVD. Follow these supplement recommendations for prevention:

Supplement	Your Daily Dosage	Comments
High-potency multivitamin/mineral with B vitamins and antioxidants	Follow label instructions.	Avoid one-a-day formulas. The most effective formulas have you taking several or more capsules/tablets a day. That's what it takes to include the many elements necessary to help protect your arteries and heart from inflammation.
Fish oil	1–2 g	Be sure that the product you take is free of contaminants.

Supplement	Your Daily Dosage	Comments
Magnesium	400 mg if not present in your multivitamin	Helps prevent the ravages of everyday stress. Keeps your artery walls relaxed.
Vitamin C	At least 500 mg if not present in your multivitamin	An important antioxidant that keeps your tissues strong, including your artery walls.
CoQ10	25–50 mg	For maximum bioavailability, choose a hydrosoluble form.

Get the Tests Done

If you have a family history of heart disease, particularly premature arterial disease (such as a sudden death before fifty or a heart attack before forty), you should undergo the entire array of blood tests we suggest in chapter 4. Thirty would be a good age to do it. If you are over thirty, then as soon as possible. Take immediate action if you have any early symptoms.

If you don't have a family history of heart disease, have the tests done when you are forty. We recommend the EBT and IMT scans (described in chapter 4) when you are fifty, but if you have a family history, premature disease, or abnormal lab tests, get them when you are forty.

Doing these screening procedures makes you an active participant in your own longevity and quality of life. You'll also help your doctor do good prevention.

What about the Genetic Factor?

Lp(a), homocysteine, and ferritin can be influenced by genetics. A predisposition to high blood pressure can be genetic. But we believe that many people use genetics as an excuse to do nothing.

If you have a father who died of a heart attack at age forty-five, does that mean you are doomed to die of a heart attack? The answer is no. The tools we now have in New Cardiology allow us to identify specific risk factors and defuse an individual's genetic minefield.

Even though you may have been dealt a susceptible set of genes, lifestyle factors are much more important. If your father was a smoker and you are not a smoker, or if you model your mother's mellow behavior rather than your father's aggressive behavior, these are modifying elements that can lower your risks.

We believe that plaque formation is really a lifestyle disease, the result of years of unhealthy eating, lack of exercise, stress, unchecked bacterial activity, and environmental toxins that conspire to damage the arteries. These factors cause inflammation—the root cause of heart disease. Our program aims to keep inflammation at bay.

Bringing Down Insulin Levels

We've spoken often about the dangers of elevated insulin and insulin resistance. Doctors use either a fasting plasma glucose test or an oral glucose tolerance test to detect insulin resistance. Both require that you fast overnight. If you have an insulin level higher than 17 µ/L, you need to take action. Fortunately, some of our favorite supplements, as mentioned in the interventions table on p. 214, help restore normal insulin function. A diet that avoids insulin-spiking foods (see chapter 9) and regular exercise (chapter 10) also help the cause. Losing just a modest amount of weight (5 to 10 percent of total body weight) through diet and moderate exercise—such as walking thirty minutes a day, five days a week—can make a big difference in preventing the ravages and progression of insulin resistance.

What to Do for Thick Blood and Iron Overload

Viscosity relates to a physical property of blood: its thickness and stickiness, factors that determine the flow rate within the circulatory system. Interactions between the flow and the protective mechanisms operating inside arterial tissue are becoming increasingly understood. Blood viscosity, an overlooked element in blood tests, is being seen, in fact, as a new major marker for identifying patients at risk for atherosclerosis.

Cardiologists, including us, have started to use a new, advanced in-office diagnostic device called a Rheolog that measures the thickness of a patient's blood, enhancing the ability to assess vulnerability for forming blood clots. A small amount of blood is taken from the patient. The device analyzes the blood and within three minutes returns a thickness number, called a thrombogenic potential.

If your cardiologist doesn't have the Rheolog yet, you can contact Rheologics Inc. (610-524-6022), the Pennsylvania medical research company that developed the device and find out if the test is administered near you. For additional contact information, see the appendix.

In the meantime, why not donate blood? You'll be helping others as you reduce your cardiac risk, lower blood viscosity, and prevent iron overload.

Who should give blood? Provided you are not iron deficient or anemic, there are no side effects from giving blood. To lower blood viscosity and protect against iron overload, it makes sense for everyone over age fifty to give blood one to four times per year. But men can start at thirty. Give blood often enough to keep your ferritin level at 100 µg/ml or lower.

If you have moderate to advanced coronary artery disease, donations will help thin down your blood. Donating periodically may be the single most important thing you can do to prevent a heart attack.

Too Much Iron? Give Blood

One of Dr. Roberts's patients had all his conventional risk factors under control. However, the man had an exceptionally high ferritin level, so Dr. Roberts recommended donating blood three times a year. The patient found out that the Red Cross in his area does not accept blood for its blood bank if blood giving is part of a medical therapy and the donor is taking multiple medications. However, for a fee, the organization will draw and discard one unit of blood. Such practices, by the way, vary across the country according to local regulations.

In this case, the particular patient had limited income. He could not afford the $50 fee. On his behalf, Dr. Roberts asked his health insurance company to cover the fee because of the risk for a heart attack. The company turned down the request.

Soon afterward, the patient suffered a nonfatal heart attack. His ferritin level had remained high, producing excessive free radical damage, and his coronary artery disease had progressed.

Five days in the hospital, a coronary angiogram, and the seven weeks of additional treatment required to stabilize his symptoms cost about $25,000. A few blood-removal sessions at $50 each probably would have prevented this unfortunate event.

Here's what else you can do to decrease your iron level:

- Cut iron consumption. Red meat is loaded with iron. Avoid iron-fortified grains and cereals.

- Toss your multivitamin/mineral supplement if it contains iron.

- Don't use iron cookware.

- Don't take more than 500 mg of vitamin C each day until your ferritin level has fallen. This otherwise wonderful vitamin can promote iron absorption.

- Check your water supply, which may be high in iron. Consider using a water filter to eliminate excess iron.

Hormones for Your Heart

The hormone system that orchestrates the countless chemical interactions inside our bodies takes a big hit as we age. Hormone output slowly but steadily drops, including the sex hormones estrogen and testosterone. Their particular decline goes far beyond sexuality, because in the highly complex world of hormones, estrogen and testosterone contribute a good deal of protection to the cardiovascular system. For both men and women, this loss of protection is, in fact, a risk factor for CVD.

Testosterone: Solid scientific evidence exists that a healthy level protects the heart in many ways. It decreases clotting tendencies, fibrinogen, Lp(a), triglycerides, blood pressure, and abdominal fat. At the same time, it promotes endothelial relaxation, HDL activity, regulation of inflammatory substances, blood sugar control, and glucose entry into cells (thus reducing insulin resistance). Testosterone's potential remains largely neglected, an underemployed method of treatment within the medical establishment.

Estrogen: A healthy level of estrogen protects women by combating free radical activity and LDL oxidation, helping keep blood sugar, Lp(a), and clotting activity in check. It also promotes HDL cholesterol, blood flow, and arterial elasticity, flexibility, and dilation. The history of hormone replacement for women has been a roller-coaster ride of tremendous promise followed by nosedives of disappointment as new risks and side effects emerge, leaving women generally confused and fearful. The field of cardiology now stands opposed to hormone replacement therapy, the common medical practice to relieve menopause discomfort until recently. This position followed the 2003 publication in the *New England*

Journal of Medicine with startling data from a major women's study. The data showed that the widely prescribed combination of chemicalized estrogen and progestin (the hormonal drug substitutes) medication may *increase* the risk of coronary artery disease. In the analysis of the data, these compounds created a 24 percent overall increase in the risk, including an 81 percent increased risk in the first year after starting the therapy.

Hormone therapy has obvious benefits but is extremely complex and must be conducted with an individualized approach under the supervision of an experienced physician. It is beyond the scope of this book to adequately cover this issue.

The standard "hormones" prescribed by most doctors are potent synthetic pharmaceutical drugs with frequent side effects and real dangers.

When appropriate, we only prescribe natural (bioidentical) hormones in our practices. They are exact chemical replicas of hormones that the body produces. Scientists have discovered how to chemically extract them from plant sources and process them into hormone preparations readily absorbed and utilized in the body. Such natural hormones are widely available today by prescription through compounding pharmacies.

Bioidentical hormones offer men and women an appealing, nonpharmaceutical option that can reduce the potential for adverse effects. Replacement therapy of this type is frequently offered by physicians specializing in antiaging medicine. For a list of such doctors, visit the Web site of the American Academy of Anti-Aging Medicine (www.world health.net/) or call their headquarters in Chicago at (773) 528-1000.

For more information on women, hormones, and cardiovascular health, you may want to obtain a copy of Dr. Sinatra's *Heart Sense for Women*.

Oral Hygiene

Over the last decade, researchers have associated the bacteria and inflammation of periodontal infections (common gum diseases) with arterial inflammation. The connection is simple: pathogenic (disease causing) bacteria migrate into the circulatory system and contribute to inflammation in the arteries. Thus, to help put out the fire in your arteries, you need to put out the fire in your mouth.

We believe, in fact, that good oral hygiene is more important than lowering cholesterol. If you clean up the bacterial act in your mouth, signs of CVD disease, such as CRP level, go down. That means there's less inflammation in your system from top to bottom.

For advice on highly effective measures you can do on your own to counteract bacterial infections of the mouth, we consulted Paul H. Keyes, a now retired researcher whose landmark investigations years ago at the National Institute of Dental Research helped to prove that both cavities and gum diseases are chronic bacterial infections. First and foremost, says Keyes, periodontal infections in adults can be prevented and mild infections can be controlled by careful dental self-care (oral hygiene) with such inexpensive and natural products as salt, baking soda, hydrogen peroxide, and apple cider vinegar. These substances are potent bacterial killers. "In sufficient quantity, they instantly kill many of the microorganisms associated with gum infections on contact," said Keyes.

Keyes has seen the killing effect repeatedly under the microscope and has recommended to many patients that they use these substances to brush as a method to arrest disease. They surpass the antibacterial potential of many toothpastes hands down, he said. Although some commercial toothpastes contain baking soda, very few pack a high enough concentration to be of any therapeutic value.

"One very easy and effective method is to first dip your toothbrush in hydrogen peroxide and then in baking soda," said Keyes.

Along with thorough brushing, oral irrigation of the mouth is another excellent way to remove food residues and reduce disease-causing germs attached to tooth surfaces. A variety of good countertop and portable irrigators are widely available, including Hydrofloss (www.hydrofloss.com) and ViaJet (www.oratec.com).

An individual with advanced gum infection needs to see a clinician who can disinfect the root surfaces and deep pockets and also provide guidance on anti-infective self-care. Many general dentists refer such patients to a periodontist, a specialist trained to treat gum disease by scaling bacterial biofilms (plaque) and calcified remains (tartar) and surgically removing infected pockets.

Lamentably, said Keyes, "conventional surgical programs often fail to eliminate bacterial infections, and the accompanying inflammatory and immune reactions may destroy so much soft tissue and bone that teeth are lost."

In 1975, Keyes began reporting on the success of a nonsurgical, anti-infective therapy he developed for severely infected gums. Among the techniques in his approach is a demonstration of the live infection via a TV system attached to a microscope. The anti-infective measures also include local treatment of infected sites with antiseptics and instruments to disinfect pockets and root surfaces, and careful training of patients in effective self-care. To find a dentist near you who uses this method, visit the Web site of the International Dental Health Foundation (members.aol.com/idhf/) or www.drpaulhkeyes.com. When you call, be sure to confirm that the dentist uses nonsurgical anti-infective periodontal therapy.

Finally, don't forget our heart-friendly supplement CoQ10. It is also excellent for combating gum disease. Those with gum disease will benefit dramatically by taking 300 mg daily. And don't forget the other supplements as well, such as vitamin C and fish oil, which can also help keep the immune system strong and reduce oral inflammation.

Nixing Nanobacteria

We think that cardiology will soon take up the challenge of nanobacteria—the miniscule microbes 1/1000th the size of other bacteria. Finnish experts believe that this insidious microorganism causes the calcification present in diseased arteries. They are refining a treatment method aimed at killing the bacteria and decalcifying the arteries. We have used it and seen patients improve and arterial calcium scores fall dramatically. This is a new CVD therapy that needs further refinement, but pilot studies in the United States and around the world have been positive.

Unfortunately, no reliable test exists at the current time to determine the presence of nanobacteria in the body. That will come as well. Treatment involves the use of EDTA, a synthetic amino acid that breaks down the calcific nanobacteria shell, along with the antibiotic tetracycline.

For more information, read *The Calcium Bomb* by science writers Douglas Mulhall and Katja Hansen. You can visit the Web site of the Nanobac Laboratory (located in Tampa, Florida) at www.nanobac.com. An extensive discussion on nanobacteria and the therapy program can also be found on Dr. Roberts's Web site www.heartfixer.com.

The Crystal Ball

We see an exciting time ahead for cardiology because so many new tools and so much new information are constantly emerging. The day is coming when no one will have to die from arterial disease.

But even today we can put out the flames of arterial disease with the best that alternative and conventional medicine has to offer. We can now determine the presence of nasty constituents within the blood—such as toxic metals—that poison the arteries. We can determine with new imaging technology the extent of a patient's calcification and whether hard plaque or soft plaque is building up.

We are beginning to utilize genetics to hone in on a patient's specific weaknesses and map out individualized remedies. One day soon, we will be able to genetically test babies shortly after birth and determine enzyme deficiencies that may set them up for heart disease forty years later. The genetic age in medicine is coming.

Soon we expect to be able to monitor endothelial function and check on the status of this critical one-cell layer that lines the arterial walls of the body. In the not-too-distant future, we may even have vaccines against atherosclerosis.

We see metabolic cardiology, electromagnetic frequency devices, and other forms of energy medicine getting noninvasively to the heart of the matter, raising ATP and rejuvenating failing hearts.

The future of cardiology isn't just about applying high-tech gadgetry and research. Arterial and cardiac health still require that patients do their share, applying the low-tech (and low-cost) healing power of diet, nutritional supplements, and lifestyle changes. These are the basics that benefit not only the cardiovascular system but the body as a whole. We are often amazed at how, in the shadow of high-tech medicine, we consistently achieve powerful healing effects with our patients by using simple, standard nutrients like vitamins E and niacin and CoQ10 and fish oil. Now we are excited by the promise shown recently by vitamin K-2 for plaque reversal. Soon we both will participate in a multicenter international research project to help clarify further the potential of K-2.

The future of cardiovascular medicine and medicine in general, must integrate the principles of a holistic approach that seeks to correct underlying causes with those of conventional medicine that addresses acute problems. There has been too much antagonism in medicine for too long—sort of like a two-party system where one side tries to beat down the other side. We have experienced this directly, and we don't like it. It's counterproductive to the interests of patients.

Fortunately, the bitterness and badmouthing seem to be receding. We give lectures at alternative medicine meetings on how alternative patients can benefit from angioplasty and bypass surgery when and if it is appropriate for them. And our mainstream cardiology journals have opened their pages to nutritional interventions.

For the sake of our patients and the economics of medicine, the future must bring about a union in which there will be no separate alternative medicine and conventional medicine. Instead, we must have smart medicine in which physicians consider combinations of nutrition, lifestyle, pharmacology, and surgery to prevent or treat CVD. Hopefully, this union will occur in time to help you and your family, and before our expensive disease management approach bankrupts the Medicare and Medicaid programs.

APPENDIX A

Resources

The seismic changes in today's health care delivery systems dictate that you take increasing responsibility for your own health and participate in decisions about your health care. It is vital that you find a knowledgeable, open-minded practitioner who will work with you to determine the safest and most effective treatments for your specific condition or prevention strategies to optimize your health.

Unfortunately, nutritional supplements and natural remedies are almost totally neglected in medical school. Thus, conventional practitioners generally lack awareness of complementary therapies, even though such therapies can be just as effective as prescription drugs.

We wish there were many cardiologists in the country practicing the way we do—that is, integrating both conventional and natural treatments in a safe and effective way to maximize patient health. At this time, our numbers are few, but interest is growing in our field. We believe that many more doctors will gravitate to this common-sense approach in the future. It works too well to be ignored.

Following are the names of cardiologists, including ourselves, who practice integrative cardiology—the New Cardiology.

Doctors Who Practice Integrative Cardiology

Lee Cowden, M.D., F.A.C.C.
6387B Camp Bowie Boulevard,
    Suite 293
Fort Worth, TX 76116
(817) 441-2504

Richard Delany, M.D., F.A.C.C.
2 Reedsdale Road
Milton, MA 02186
(617) 698-0715

Stephen Devries, M.D., F.A.C.C.
Medical Director, University of
    Illinois Healthy Heart Center

Lake Cook Plaza
405 Lake Cook Road, Suite A205
Deerfield, IL 60015
(847) 272-8500
www.healthyheartcenter.com

Howard Elkin, M.D., F.A.C.C.
HeartWise Fitness and Longevity
   Center
8135 Painter Avenue, Suite 204
Whittier, CA 90602
(562) 945-6693
www.heartwise.com

Peter Langsjoen, M.D., F.A.C.C.,
   P.A.
1120 Medical Drive
Tyler, TX 75701
(903) 595-4962
www.coenzymeq10.org

James C. Roberts, M.D., F.A.C.C.
3110 West Central Avenue
Toledo, OH 43606
(419) 531-4235
www.heartfixer.com
www.amri-ohio.com

Marc A. Silver, M.D., F.A.C.C.
Director, Heart Failure Institute
University of Illinois/Advocate
   Christ Medical Center
4440 W. 95th Street, Suite 319 South
Oak Lawn, IL 60453
(708) 346-4236

Stephen T. Sinatra, M.D., F.A.C.C.,
   C.N.S., C.B.T.
Preventive & Metabolic Cardiology
257 East Center Street
Manchester, CT 06040
(860) 643-5101
www.drsinatra.com

Cardiovascular Surgeons

Gerald Lemole, M.D., F.A.C.C.
4745 Ogletown Stanton Road
Medical Arts Pavilion, Suite 205
Newark, DE 19713
(302) 738-0448

Mehmet Oz, M.D., F.A.C.S.
New York Presbyterian Hospital
Milstein Hospital Building,
   Room 7 GN 43
177 Fort Washington Avenue
New York, NY 10032
(212) 342-5588

Frederic J. Vagnini, M.D., F.A.C.C.,
   F.A.C.S.
The Cardiovascular Wellness
   Center
1600 Stewart Avenue
Westbury, NY 11590
(516) 222-2288
www.vagnini.com

**Laboratories That Perform
Advanced Cardiology Risk
Factor Testing**

Antibody Assay Reference
   Laboratory
1715 E. Wilshire, Suite 715
Santa Ana, CA 92705
(800) 522-2611
www.antibodyassay.com

Great Smokies Diagnostic
   Laboratory
63 Zillicoa Street
Asheville, NC 28801
(800) 522-4762
www.gsdl.com/home/

Immunosciences Lab, Inc.
8693 Wilshire Boulevard,
    Suite 200
Beverly Hills, CA 90211
(800) 950-4686
www.immuno-sci-lab.com/index2
    .html

Metametrix Clinical Laboratory
4855 Peachtree Industrial
    Boulevard, Suite 201
Norcross, GA 30092
(800) 221-4640
www.metametrix.com/

AA/EPA Testing

Nutrasource Diagnostics, Inc.
Granbry Building, Suite 4
130 Research Lane
University of Guelph Research
    Park
Guelph, Ontario, Canada N1G 5G3
(877) 557-7722
www.nutrasource.ca

Your Future Health
P.O. Box 1369
Tavares, FL 32778
(877) 468-6934
www.yourfuturehealth.com

Advanced Scanning

To find a facility near you that
    performs general electric imatron
    EBT scanning, visit www
    .geimatron.com/index.html.

Blood Viscosity Testing

Rheologics, Inc.
15 East Uwchlan Avenue, Suite 414
Exton, PA 19341
(610) 524-6022
www.rheologics.com

Nanobacteria Research, Tests, and Physician Referrals

Nanobac Laboratories
2727 W. Martin Luther King
    Boulevard, Suite 850
Tampa, FL 33607
(813) 264-2241
www.nanobac.com/

Supplements

Beyond a Century
173 Lily Bay Road
Greenville, ME 04441
(800) 777-1324
www.beyond-a-century.com
For quality bulk L-arginine at a low
    price.

BioImmune, Inc.
8300 N. Hayden Road, Suite A203
Scottsdale, AZ 85258
(888) 663-8844
www.bioimmune.com
Producer of DetoxMaxPlus.

Dr. Sinatra's Advanced
    BioSolutions
7811 Montrose Road
Potomac, MD 20854
(800) 304-1708
www.drsinatra.com

Canada RNA Biochemical, Inc.
152-8211 Akroyd Road
Richmond, British Columbia,
    Canada V6X 3K8
(866) 287-4986
www.canadarna.com
Producer of lumbrokinase.

Health Science Nutrition, L.L.C.
325 Main Street
Kentlands, MD 20878
(877) 877-1970
www.hsfighters.com
To obtain Metafolin, a patented
    form of high-absorption folic
    acid, in combination with
    vitamin B-12, for homocysteine
    lowering.

Optimum Health International,
    L.L.C.
257 East Center Street
Manchester, CT 06040
(800) 228-1507
www.opthealth.com

Sigma-Tau HealthScience, Inc.
Sigma-Tau, Inc.
800 South Frederick Avenue,
    Suite 300
Gaithersburg, MD 20877
(800) 447-0169
www.sigmatau.com
Sigma-Tau provides high-quality
    L-carnitine and other carnitine
    products for pharmaceutical and
    supplement use.

Tishcon Corporation
30 New York Avenue
Westbury, NY 11590-5910
(800) 848-8442
www.tishcon.com
Producer of hydrosoluble CoQ10
    (Q-Gel).

Valen Labs, Inc.
13840 Johnson Street NE
Minneapolis, MN 55304
(763) 757-0032
www.bioenergy.com
Producer of D-ribose.

Recommended Reading

Newsletters

The *Sinatra Health Report*, a monthly newsletter covering the newest
    research and clinical advances in cardiology and general medicine, is
    available through Phillips Health LLC, 7811 Montrose Road, Potomac,
    MD 20854, (800) 211-7643. The annual subscription is $69. The report
    is dedicated to the prevention and treatment of disease.

Books

Eliot, R. S. *From Stress to Strength: How to Lighten Your Load and Save Your
    Life*. New York: Bantam, 1995.
Eliot, R. S., and D. L. Breo. *Is It Worth Dying For?* New York: Bantam,
    1984.
Mulhall, D., and K. Hansen. *The Calcium Bomb*. Cranston, RI: Writers'
    Collective, 2004.

Sears, B. *The Age-Free Zone.* New York: HarperCollins, 1999.

———. *Enter the Zone.* New York: HarperCollins, 1995.

———. *The Omega Rx Zone.* New York: HarperCollins, 2002.

Sinatra, S. T. *The Coenzyme Q10 Phenomenon.* Chicago: Keats, 1998.

———. *Heartbreak and Heart Disease.* Chicago: Keats, 1999.

———. *The Sinatra Solution.* North Bergen, NJ: Basic Health, 2005.

Sinatra, S. T., and J. Sinatra. *Lower Your Blood Pressure in Eight Weeks.* New York: Ballantine, 2003.

Sinatra, S. T., with J. Sinatra and R. J. Lieberman. *Heart Sense for Women.* New York: Penguin Putnam, 2001.

APPENDIX B

Glycemic Index of Carbohydrates

For more details on the glycemic index, visit www.glycemicindex.com.

Rapid Inducers of Insulin
Glycemic Index Greater than 100 Percent

GRAIN-BASED FOODS
Cornflakes
French bread
Instant rice
Microwaved potatoes
Millet
Puffed rice
Puffed wheat

SIMPLE SUGARS
Glucose
Maltose

SNACKS
Puffed rice cakes
Tofu ice cream

Glycemic Index between 80 and 100 Percent

GRAIN-BASED FOODS
Brown and white rice
Grapenuts
Instant mashed potatoes
Muesli
Oat bran
Rolled oats
Shredded wheat
Whole-wheat bread

VEGETABLES
Carrots
Corn
Parsnips

FRUITS
Apricots
Bananas
Mangoes
Papayas
Raisins

SNACKS
Corn chips
Ice cream (low-fat)
Rye crisps

Moderate Inducers of Insulin

Glycemic Index between 50 and 80 Percent

GRAIN-BASED FOODS
All-bran cereal
All pastas, including white and
    whole-wheat spaghetti
Pumpernickel bread

FRUITS
Oranges
Orange juice

VEGETABLES
Baked beans

Garbanzo beans (canned)
Navy beans
Peas
Pinto beans

SIMPLE SUGARS
Lactose
Sucrose

SNACKS
Candy bar*
Potato chips (with fat)*

Low Inducers of Insulin

Glycemic Index between 30 and 50 Percent

GRAIN-BASED FOODS
Barley
Oatmeal (slow-cooking)
Whole-grain rye bread

FRUITS
Apples
Apple juice
Applesauce
Grapes
Peaches
Pears

VEGETABLES
Black-eyed peas
Chickpeas
Kidney beans (dried or canned)
Lentils
Peas
Tomato soup

DAIRY PRODUCTS
Ice cream (high-fat)*
Milk (skim)
Milk (whole)*
Yogurt

Glycemic Index 30 Percent or Less

FRUITS
Cherries
Grapefruits
Plums

VEGETABLES
Soy beans

SNACKS
Peanuts*

*High-fat content slows the rate of absorption of carbohydrates into the body.

Selected Scientific References

Abbott, R. D, F. Ando, K. H. Masaki, et al. Dietary magnesium intake and the future risk of coronary heart disease (the Honolulu Heart Program). *Am J Cardiol* 2003;92(6):665–9.

Al-Delaimy, W. K., E. B. Rimm, W. C. Willett, et al. Magnesium intake and risk of coronary heart disease among men. *J Am Coll Nutr* 2004;23(1):63–70.

Arita, M., F. Bianchini, and J. Aliberti. Stereochemical assignment, antiinflammatory properties, and receptor for the omega-3 lipid mediator resolvin E1. *J Exp Med* 2004;201(5):713–22.

Aviram, M., M. Rosenblat, D. Gaitini, et al. Pomegranate juice consumption for 3 years by patients with carotid artery stenosis reduces common carotid intima-media thickness, blood pressure and LDL oxidation. *Clin Nutr* 2004;23:423–33.

Barzi, F., M. Woodward, R. M. Marfisi, et al. Mediterranean diet and all-causes mortality after myocardial infarction: results from the GISSI-Prevenzione trial. *Eur J Clin Nutr* 2003;57(4):604–11.

Berk, L. S., D. L. Felten, S. A. Tan, et al. Modulation of neuroimmune parameters during the eustress of humor-associated mirthful laughter. *Altern Ther Health Med* 2001;7(2):62–76.

Berman, M., A. Erman, T. Ben-Gal, et al. Coenzyme Q10 in patients with end-stage heart failure awaiting cardiac transplantation: a randomized, placebo-controlled study. *Clin Cardiol* 2004;27(10):A26.

Boger, R. H., S. M. Bode-Boger, R. P. Brandes, et al. Dietary L-arginine reduces the progression of atherosclerosis in cholesterol-fed rabbits. *Circulation* 1997;96:1282–90.

Bostrom, K. Insights into the mechanism of vascular calcification. *Am J Cardiol* 2001;88(2-A):20E–22E.

Brambel, C. E. The role of flavonoids in Coumadin anticoagulant therapy. *Ann NY Acad Sci* 1955;61(3):678–83.

Brault, J. J., and R. L. Terjung. Purine salvage to adenine nucleotides in different skeletal muscle fiber types. *J Appl Physiol* 2001;91:231–8.

Bruno, R. S., R. Ramakrishnan, T. J. Montine, et al. α-Tocopherol disappearance is faster in cigarette smokers and is inversely related to their ascorbic acid status. *Am J Clin Nutr* 2005;81(1):95–103.

Budoff, M. J., J. Takasu, F. R. Flores, et al. Inhibiting progression of coronary calcification using aged garlic extract in patients receiving statin therapy: a preliminary study. *Prev Med* 2004;39(5):985–91.

Carlson, L. A. Nicotinic acid: the broad-spectrum lipid drug. A 50th anniversary review. *J Intern Med* 2005;258(2):94–114.

Cavallini, G., S. Caracciolo, G. Vitali, et al. Carnitine versus androgen administration in the treatment of sexual dysfunction, depressed mood, and fatigue associated with male aging. *Urology* 2004;63(4):641–6.

Cesarone, M. R., G. Belcaro, A. N. Nicolaides, et al. Prevention of venous thrombosis in long-haul flights with Flite Tabs: the LONFLIT-FLITE randomized, controlled trial. *Angiology* 2003;54(5):531–9.

Chan, K., A. Oza, and L. Siu. The statins as anticancer agents. *Clin Cancer Res* 2003;9(1):10–19.

Chopra, R. K., R. Goldman, S. T. Sinatra, et al. Relative bioavailability of coenzyme Q10 formulations in human subjects. *Int J Vitam Nutr Res* 1998;68(2):109–13.

Clark, A., A. Seidler, and M. Miller. Inverse association between sense of humor and coronary heart disease. *Int J Cardiol* 2001;80(1):87–8.

Colonna, P., and S. Iliceto. Myocardial infarction and left ventricular remodeling: results of the CEDIM trial. Carnitine Ecocardiografia Digitalizzata Infarto Miocardico. *Am Heart J* 2000;139(2 Pt 3):S124–30.

Cooke, J. P., A. H. Singer, P. Tsao, et al. Antiatherogenic effects of L-arginine in the hypercholesterolemic rabbit. *J Clin Invest* 1992;90: 1168–72.

Cutler, P. Deferoxamine therapy in high-ferritin diabetes. *Diabetes* 1989; 38:1207–10.

Debaberata, M., and J. Yadav. Carotid artery intimal-medial thickness: indicator of atherosclerotic burden and response to risk factor modification. *Am Heart J* 2002;114:753–9.

De Lorgeril, M., P. Salen, J. L. Martin, et al. Mediterranean diet, traditional risk factors, and the rate of cardiovascular complications after myocardial infarction: final report of the Lyon Diet Heart Study. *Circulation* 1999; 99:779–85.

De Nigris, F., S. Williams-Ignarro, L. O. Lerman, et al. Beneficial effects of pomegranate juice on oxidation-sensitive genes and endothelial nitric oxide synthase activity at sites of perturbed shear stress. *Proc Natl Acad Sci USA* 2005;102(13):4896–901.

Dhore, C. R., J. P. Cleutjens, E. Lutgens, et al. Differential expression of bone matrix regulatory proteins in human atherosclerotic plaques. *Arterioscler Thromb Vasc Biol* 2001;21(12):1998–2003.

Duffy, S. J., E. S. Biegelsen, M. Holbrook, et al. Iron chelation improves endothelial function in patients with coronary artery disease. *Circulation* 2001;103(23):2799–804.

Erkkila, A.T., A. H. Lichtenstein, D. Mozaffarian, et al. Fish intake is associated with a reduced progression of coronary artery atherosclerosis in postmenopausal women with coronary artery disease. *Am J Clin Nutr* 2004;80:626–32.

Ferrara, L. A., A. S. Raimondi, L. D'Episcopo, et al. Olive oil and reduced need for antihypertensive medications. *Arch Intern Med* 2000;160:837–42.

Festa, A., R. D'Agostino, R. P. Tracy, et al. Elevated levels of acute-phase proteins and plasminogen activator inhibitor-1 predict the development of type 2 diabetes. The Insulin Resistance Atherosclerosis Study. *Diabetes* 2002;5:1131–7.

Fletcher, R. H., and K. M. Fairfield. Vitamins for chronic disease prevention in adults. *JAMA* 2002;287:3127–9.

Folkers, K., P. Langsjoen, and P. H. Langsjoen. Therapy with coenzyme Q10 of patients in heart failure who are eligible or ineligible for a transplant. *Biochem Biophys Res Commun* 1992;182(1):247–53.

Folkers, K., P. Lansgsjoen, R. Willis, et al. Lovastatin decreases coenzyme Q levels in humans. *Proc Natl Acad Sci USA* 1990;87:8931–4.

Forman, J. P., E. B. Rimm, M. J. Stampfer, et al. Folate intake and the risk of incident hypertension among US women. *JAMA* 2005;293(3):320–9.

Forrester, J. S. Prevention of plaque rupture: a new paradigm of therapy. *Ann Intern Med* 2002;137(10):823–33.

Frustaci, A. Marked elevation of myocardial trace elements in idiopathic dilated cardiomyopathy compared with secondary cardiac dysfunction. *J Am Coll Cardiol* 1999;33:1578–83.

Gallo, L. C., W. M. Troxel, L. H. Kuller, et al. Marital status, marital quality, and atherosclerotic burden in postmenopausal women. *Psychosom Med* 2003;65(6):952–62.

Glurich, I., S. Grossi, B. Albini, et al. Systemic inflammation in cardiovascular and periodontal disease: comparative study. *Clin Diag Lab Immun* 2002;9(2):425–32.

Graham, D. J., J. A. Staffa, D. Shantin, et al. Incidence of hospitalized rhabdomyolysis in patients treated with lipid-lowering drugs. *JAMA* 2004; 292(21):2585–90.

Graham, I. M. Plasma homocysteine as a risk factor for vascular disease. The European Concerted Action Project. *JAMA* 1997;277:1775–81.

Greenland, P., J. Abrams, G. P. Aurigemma, et al. Beyond secondary prevention: identifying the high-risk patient for primary prevention: noninvasive tests of atherosclerotic burden. *Circulation* 2000;101:E16–22.

Guallar, E. Mercury, fish oils, and the risk of myocardial infarction. *N Engl J Med* 2002;347:1747–54.

Hadj, A., S. Pepe, F. Rosenfeldt, et al. Preoperative preparation for cardiac surgery utilizing a combination of metabolic, physical and mental therapy. In press.

Haffner, S. M. Insulin resistance, inflammation, and the prediabetic state. *Am J Cardiol* 2003;92(4A):18J–26J.

Hanna, F. W. F., and B. G. Issa. Hyperlipidaemia and cardiovascular disease: C-reactive protein and atherosclerosis—new dimensions. *Curr Opin Lipidol* 2002;13(1):101–3.

Harris, T. B., L. Ferrucci, R. P. Tracy, et al. Associations of elevated interleukin-6 and C-reactive protein levels with mortality in the elderly. *Am J Med* 1999;106:506–12.

Heber, D. Vegetables, fruits and phytoestrogens in the prevention of diseases. *J Postgrad Med* 2004;50(2):145–9.

Heeschen, C., C. W. Hamm, U. Laufs, et al. Withdrawal of statins increases event rates in patients with acute coronary syndromes. *Circulation* 2002;105:1446–52.

Holmquist, C., S. Larsson, A. Wolk, et al. Multivitamin supplements are inversely associated with risk of myocardial infarction in men and women—Stockholm Heart Epidemiology Program (SHEEP). *J Nutr* 2003;133(8):2650–4.

Horne, B. D., J. B. Muhlestein, J. F. Carlquist, et al. Statin therapy, lipid levels, C-reactive protein, and the survival of patients with angiographically severe coronary artery disease. *J Am Coll Cardiol* 2000;36:1774–80.

Januzzi, J. L., and R. C. Pasternak. Depression, hostility, and social isolation in patients with coronary artery disease. *Curr Treat Options Cardiovasc Med* 2002;4(1):77–85.

Jin, L., H. Jin, G. Zhang, et al. Changes in coagulation and tissue plasminogen activator after the treatment of cerebral infarction with lumbrokinase. *Clin Hemorheol Microcirc* 2000;23(2-4):213–8.

Judy, W. V., W. W. Stogsdill, and K. Folkers. Myocardial preservation by therapy with coenzyme Q10 during heart surgery. *Clin Investig* 1993;71(8 Suppl):S155–61.

Kajander, O., and N. Ciftcioglu. Nanobacteria: an alternative mechanism for pathogenic intra- and extra-cellular calcification and stone formation. *Proc Natl Acad Sci USA* 1998;95:8274–9.

Kessler, C., C. Spitzer, D. Stauske, et al. The apolipoprotein E and beta-fibrinogen G/A-455 gene polymorphisms are associated with ischemic stroke involving large-vessel disease. *Arterioscler Thromb Vasc Biol* 1997;17(11):2880–4.

Knekt, P., J. Ritz, M. Pereira, et al. Antioxidant vitamins and coronary heart disease risk: a pooled analysis of 9 cohorts. *Am J Clin Nutr* 2004;80:1508–20.

Kolovou, G., D. Daskalova, and D. P. Mikhailidis. Apolipoprotein E polymorphism and atherosclerosis. *Angiology* 2003;54(1):59–71.

Konishi, M., H. Iso, Y. Komachi, et al. Associations of serum total cholesterol, different types of stroke, and stenosis distribution of cerebral arteries. The Akita Pathology Study. *Stroke* 1993;24:954–64.

Korrick, S. A., D. J. Hunter, A. Rotnitzky, et al. Lead and hypertension in a sample of middle-aged women. *Am J Public Health* 1999;89:330–5.

Koscielny, J., D. Klussendorf, R. Latza, et al. The antiatherosclerotic effect of *Allium sativum*. *Atherosclerosis* 2000;150(2):437–8.

Koton, S., D. Tanne, N. M. Bornstein, et al. Triggering risk factors for ischemic stroke: A case-crossover study. *Neurology* 2004;63:2006–10.

Labiche, L. A., W. Chan, K. R. Saldin, et al. Sex and acute stroke presentation. *Ann Emer Med* 2002;40(5):453–60.

Langsjoen, P., and P. H. Langsjoen. Treatment of essential hypertension with CoQ10. *Mol Aspects Med* 1994(15 suppl):S265–72.

Langsjoen, P. H., and A. M. Langsjoen. Overview of the use of CoQ10 in cardiovascular disease. *Biofactors* 1999;9(2–4):273–84.

Lepor, N. E., H. Madyoon, and G. Friede. The emerging use of 16- and 64-slice computed tomography coronary angiography in clinical cardiovascular practice. *Rev Cardiovasc Med* 2005;6(1):47–53.

Lesser, M. Testosterone propionate therapy in one hundred cases of angina pectoris. *J Clin Endocrinol* 1946;6:549–57.

Li, J. J., and J. L. Chen. Inflammation may be a bridge connecting hypertension and atherosclerosis. *Med Hypotheses* 2005;64(5):925–9.

Liao, J. Isoprenoids as mediators of the biological effects of statins. *J Clin Invest* 2002;110(3):285–8.

Lio, D., L. Scola, A. Crivello, et al. Inflammation, genetics and longevity: further studies on the protective effects in men of IL-10-1082 promoter SNP and its interaction with TNF-308 promoter SNP. *J Med Genet* 2003;40:296–9.

Mangoni, A. A., R. A. Sherwood, C. G. Swift, et al. Folic acid enhances endothelial function and reduces blood pressure in smokers: a randomized controlled trial. *J Intern Med* 2002;252(6):497–503.

McCully, K. *The Heart Revolution: The Extraordinary Discovery That Finally Laid the Cholesterol Myth to Rest.* New York: Perennial Currents, 2000.

———. Homocysteine and vascular disease. *Nat Med* 1996;2:386–9.

McFarlane, S., R. Muniyappa, R. Francisco, et al. Pleiotropic effects of statins: lipid reduction and beyond. *J Clin Endocrinol Metab* 2002;87(4):1451–58.

McGill, H. C., Jr., C. A. McMahan, A. W. Zieske, et al. Association of coronary heart disease risk factors with microscopic qualities of coronary atherosclerosis in youth. *Circulation* 2000;102:374–9.

Meigs, J. B., F. B. Hu, N. Rifai, et al. Biomarkers of endothelial dysfunction and risk of type 2 diabetes mellitus. *JAMA* 2004;291:1978–86.

Meyer, F., I. Bairati, and G. R. Dagenais. Lower ischemic heart disease incidence and mortality among vitamin supplement users. *Can J Cardiol* 1996;12(10):930–4.

Miller, K. L., R. S. Liebowitz, L. K. Newby, et al. Complementary and alternative medicine in cardiovascular disease: a review of biologically based approaches. *Am Heart J* 2004:401–11.

Mitka, M. Researchers examine effects of dietary magnesium on type II diabetes risk. *JAMA* 2004;291(9):1056–7.

Molyneux, S., C. Florkowski, M. Lever, et al. The bioavailability of coenzyme Q10 supplements available in New Zealand differs markedly. *NZ Med J* 2004;117(1203):U1108.

Nash, R. A. The biomedical ethics of alternative, complementary, and integrative medicine. *Altern Ther* 1999;5:92–5.

Nissen, S. E., S. J. Nicholls, I. Sipahi, et al. Effect of very high-intensity statin therapy on regression of coronary atherosclerosis. The ASTEROID Trial. *JAMA* 2006;295(13):1556–65.

No author. Influence of adherence to treatment and response of cholesterol on mortality in the coronary drug project. *N Engl J Med* 1980;303(18):1038–41.

Nygard, O., J. E. Nordrehaug, H. Refsum, et al. Plasma homocysteine levels and mortality in patients with coronary artery disease. *N Engl J Med* 1997;337(4):230–6.

Ornish, D., L. Scherwitz, J. Billings, et al. Can intensive lifestyle changes reverse coronary heart disease? Five-year follow-up of the Lifestyle Heart Trial. *JAMA* 1998;280:2001–7.

Paterson, J. C. Some factors in the causation of intimal hemorrhages and in the precipitation of coronary thrombi. *Can Med Assoc J* 1941; 44:114–20.

Pliml, W., T. von Arnim, A. Stablein, et al. Effects of ribose on exercise-induced ischemia in stable coronary artery disease. *Lancet* 1992;340:507–10.

Raggi, P. The use of electron-beam computed tomography as a tool for primary prevention. *Am J Cardiol* 2001;88(7B):28J–32J.

Rapola, J. M., J. Virtamo, S. Ripatti, et al. Effects of alpha-tocopherol and beta-carotene supplements on symptoms, progression, and prognosis of angina pectoris. *Heart* 1998;79:454–8.

Rich, S., and V. V. McLaughlin. Detective of subclinical cardiovascular disease: the emerging role of electron-beam computed tomography. *Prev Med* 2002;34(1):1–10.

Ridker, P. M., C. H. Hennekens, J. E. Buring, et al. C-reactive protein and other markers of inflammation in the prediction of cardiovascular disease in women. *N Engl J Med* 2000;342(12):836–43.

Ridker, P. M., J. E. Manson, J. E. Buring, et al. Homocysteine and risk of cardiovascular disease among post-menopausal women. *JAMA* 1999; 281(19):1817–21.

Rosenfeldt, F., F. Miller, P. Nagley, et al. Response of the senescent heart to stress: clinical therapeutic strategies and quest for mitochondrial predictors of biological age. *Ann NY Acad Sci* 2004;1019:78–84.

Salonen, J. T. High stored iron levels are associated with excess risk of myocardial infarction in eastern Finnish men. *Circulation* 1992;86:803–11.

———. Intake of mercury from fish, lipid peroxidation, and the risk of myocardial infarction and coronary, cardiovascular, and any death in eastern Finnish men. *Circulation* 1995;91:645–55.

———. Mercury accumulation and accelerated progression of carotid atherosclerosis: a population-based prospective 4-year follow-up study in men in eastern Finland. *Atheroslcerosis* 2000;148:265–73.

Schnyder, G., M. Roffi, Y. Flammer, et al. Effect of homocysteine-lowering therapy with folic acid, vitamin B_{12}, and vitamin B_6 on clinical outcome after percutaneous coronary intervention: the Swiss Heart Study: a randomized controlled trial. *JAMA* 2002;288:973–9.

Schulman, S. P., L. C. Becker, D. A. Kass, et al. L-arginine therapy in acute myocardial infarction: the Vascular Interaction with Age in Myocardial Infarction (VINTAGE MI) randomized clinical trial. *JAMA* 2006; 295:58–64.

Shechter, M., C. N. Bairey Merz, H. Stuehlinger, et al. Effects of oral magnesium therapy on exercise tolerance, exercise-induced chest pain, and quality of life in patients with coronary artery disease. *Am J Cardiol* 2003;91(5):517–21.

Seelig, M. S. Consequences of magnesium deficiency on the enhancement of stress reactions; preventive and therapeutic implications. *J Am Coll Nutr* 1994;13(5):429–46.

Selhub, J., P. F. Jacques, P. W. Wilson, et al. Vitamin status and intake as primary determinants of homocysteinemia in an elderly population. *JAMA* 1993;270(22):2693–8.

Seppanen, K., P. Soininen, J. T. Salonen, et al. Does mercury promote lipid peroxidation? An in vitro study concerning mercury, copper, and iron in peroxidation of low-density lipoprotein. *Biol Trace Elem Res* 2004; 101(2):117–32.

Sheffield, M. C. Multiple effects of statins in nonlipid disease states. *US Pharm* 2004;29:38–54.

Shiplak, M. G. Estrogen and progestin, lipoprotein(a), and the risk of recurrent coronary heart disease events after menopause. *JAMA* 2000; 283:1845–52.

Siegel, G., F. Michel, M. Ploch, et al. Inhibition of arteriosclerotic plaque development by garlic. *Wien Med Wochenschr* 2004;154(21–22):515–22.

Silver, M. A., P. H. Langsjoen, S. Szabo, et al. Effect of Atorvastatin on left ventricular diastolic function and ability of coenzyme Q10 to reverse that dysfunction. *Am J Cardiol* 2004;94:1306–10.

Sinatra, S. T. Coenzyme Q10: a vital therapeutic nutrient for the heart with special application in congestive heart failure. *Conn Med* 1997; 61(11):707–11.

————. Refractory congestive heart failure successfully managed with high dose coenzyme Q10 administration. *Mol Aspects Med* 1997; 18(Suppl):S299–305.

————. Alternative medicine for the conventional cardiologist. *Heart Dis* 2000;2(1):16–30.

————. Coenzyme Q10 and congestive heart failure. *Ann Intern Med* 2000;133(9):745–6.

————. Is cholesterol lowering with statins the gold standard for treating patients with cardiovascular risk and disease? *South Med J* 2003; 93(3):220–2.

Sinatra, S. T., and J. DeMarco. Free radicals, oxidative stress, oxidized low density lipoprotein (LDL), and the heart: antioxidants and other strategies to limit cardiovascular damage. *Conn Med* 1995;59(10):579–88.

Sinatra, S. T., W. H. Frishman, S. J. Peterson, et al. Cardiovascular pharmacotherapeutics. In *Use of Alternatiave/Complementary Medicine in Treating Cardiovascular Disease*, ed. W. H. Frishman and W. Sonenblick. New York: McGraw-Hill Medical Publishing Division, 2003, pp. 857–74.

Singh, R. B., G. S. Wander, A. Rastogi, et al. Randomized, double-blind placebo-controlled trial of coenzyme Q10 in patients with acute myocardial infarction. *Cardiovasc Drugs Ther* 1998;12(4):347–53.

Siscovick, D. S., T. E. Raghunathan, I. King, et al. Dietary intake and cell membrane levels of long-chain n-3 polyunsaturated fatty acids and the risk of primary cardiac arrest. *JAMA* 1995;274:1363–7.

Spieker, L. E., D. Hurlimann, and F. Ruschitzka. Mental stress induces prolonged endothelial dysfunction via endothelin-A receptors. *Circulation* 2002;105(24):2817–20.

Stone, N. J. The Gruppo Italiano per lo Studio della Sopravvivenza nell'Infarto Miocardio (GISSI) Prevenzione. Trial on fish oil and vitamin E supplementation in myocardial infarction survivors. *Curr Cardiol Rep* 2000;2(5):445–51.

Sumner, M. D., E. Eller, and G. Weidner. Effective pomegranate juice consumption on mild cardioperfusion in patients with coronary heart disease. *Am J Cardiol* 2005;96:810–4.

Takase, B., H. Etsuda, Y. Matsushima, et al. Effect of chronic oral supplementation with vitamins on the endothelial function in chronic smokers. *Angiology* 2004;55(6):653–60.

Tan, S. A., L. G. Tan, L. S. Berk, et al. Mirthful laughter an effective adjunct in cardiac rehabilitation. *Can J Cardiol* 1997;13(suppl B):190.

Thomas, S. R., P. K. Witting, and R. Stocker. A role for reduced coenzyme Q in atherosclerosis? *Biofactors* 1999;9(2-4):207–24.

Tintut, Y., and L. L. Demer. Recent advances in multifactorial regulation of vascular calcification. *Curr Opin Lipidol* 2001;12(5):555–60.

Tsaih, S. W., S. Korrick Schwartz, et al. Lead, diabetes, hypertension, and renal function: the Normative Aging Study. *Environ Health Perspect* 2004;112(11):1178–82.

Tullson, P. C., and R. L. Terjung. Adenine nucleotide synthesis in exercising and endurance-trained skeletal muscle. *Am J Physiol* 1991;261:C342–7.

Vermeulen, A. Estradiol in elderly men. *Aging Male* 2002;5(2):98–102.

Walton, K. G., R. H. Schneider, and S. Nidich. Review of controlled research on the transcendental meditation program and cardiovascular disease. Risk factors, morbidity, and mortality. *Cardiol Rev* 2004;12(5):262–6.

Wan, X. S., J. H. Ware, Z. Zhou, et al. Protection against radiation-induced oxidative stress in cultured human epithelial cells by treatment with antioxidant agents. *Int J Radiat Oncol Biol Phys* 2006;64(5):1475–81.

Watanabe, H., M. Kakihana, S. Ohtsuka, et al. Randomized, double-blind, placebo-controlled study of ascorbate on the preventive effect of nitrate tolerance in patients with congestive heart failure. *Circulation* 1998; 97:886–91.

Willis, G. C., A. W. Light, and W. S. Cow. Serial arteriography in atherosclerosis. *Can Med Assoc J* 1954;71:562–72.

Wilt, T. J., H. E. Bloomfield, R. MacDonald, et al. Effectiveness of statin therapy in adults with coronary heart disease. *Arch Intern Med* 2004;164:1427–36.

Wisloff, U., S. M. Najjar, O. Ellingsen, et al. Cardiovascular risk factors emerge after artificial selection for aerobic capacity. *Science* 2005;307(5708):334–5.

Wolfrum, S., K. Jensen, and J. Liao. Endothelium-dependent effects of statins. *Arterioscler Thromb Vas Biol* 2003;23(5):372–8.

Yokota, K., M. Kato, and F. Lister. Clinical efficacy of magnesium supplementation in patients with type II diabetes. *J Am Coll Nutr* 2004;23(5):506S–9.

Zhang, G. P., H. M. Jin, M. Zhang, et al. Anticoagulative and fibrinolytic effects of lumbrokinase and their relation to tissue plasminogen activator. *Chinese J Geriatr* 1998;6(17):366–8.

Zimmer, H. G. Regulation of and intervention into the oxidative pentose phosphate pathway and adenine nucleotide metabolism in the heart. *Mol Cell Biochem* 1996;160–1(1):101–9.

Zumoff, B. Hormonal abnormalities in obesity. *Acta Med Scand* 1988;723 (Suppl):153–60.

Index